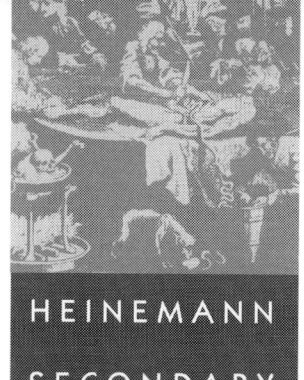

HEINEMANN

SECONDARY

HISTORY

PROJECT

MEDICINE THROUGH TIME

Bob Rees • Paul Shuter

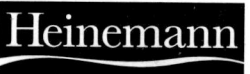

Heinemann Educational Publishers

Halley Court, Jordan Hill, Oxford OX2 8EJ
a division of Reed Educational &
Professional Publishing Ltd

OXFORD FLORENCE PRAGUE MADRID ATHENS
MELBOURNE AUCKLAND KUALA LUMPUR
SINGAPORE TOKYO PORTSMOUTH NH (USA)
CHICAGO MEXICO CITY SAO PAULO

© Bob Rees and Paul Shuter, 1996

First published 1996

00 99 98 97 96
10 9 8 7 6 5 4 3 2 1

British Library Cataloguing in Publication Data
A catalogue record for this book is available from
the British Library

ISBN 0 435 30922 6

Produced by Dennis Fairey and Associates Ltd
Cover design by The Wooden Ark Studio
Illustrated by Arthur Phillips
Printed and Bound in Spain by Mateu Cromo

Acknowledgements

The publishers would like to thank the following for permission to
reproduce copyright material:

Ancient Art and Architecture Collection: 1.1A, 5.3I Chester Beatty
Library, Dublin 7.4F Tim Beddow/Science Photo Library 12.3P
Count Robert Bégoüen, Musée Pujol, France: 1.2C Bodleian Library 8.4F
9.1A Bridgeman Art Library 2.2A British Library Reproductions 8.4G,
8.7O, 9T British Museum Library 4.6I, 9.2G Cambridge University
Library 8.2D Jean-Loup Charmet/Science Photo Library 11.4M
Coo.ee Historical Picture Archive 1.4E, 1.4F Corbis Bettmann/UPI
12.2L Francesca Countway Library 12.1C C. M. Dixon 3.1A, 3.2B,
4.1A, 5.3H E. T. Archive 4.6K, 12.1A Mary Evans Picture Library 10.1
(top box p.75), 11.1 (box p.79), 11.1C, 11.2I, 11.3 (box p. 83), 11.5
(box p.88), 12.5 (top box p. 108), 13.3(2) Alexander Fleming Laboratory
Museum, St Mary's Hospital, Paddington 11.5O, 11.5P Frank Graham
5.3G Hildesheim Museum 2.3C Michael Holford 4.3F, 5.3E, 7.2B Tim
Holt/Science Photo Library 12.3T Hulton Deutsch Collection 11.3J,
12,2 (box p.103), 12.5 (bottom box p.108), 13.2 (box p.112) Hutchinson
Library 12.3S Louvre Ager 4.7L Mansell Collection 10.1B, 12.4U, 13.1B,
13.2K Master and Fellows, Trinity College, Cambridge 8.6M Musee
Pasteur 11.3 (box p.83), 11.6(1) National Portrait Gallery, London 9
(p.72) Natural History Museum 12B Punch Library 13.2L, 13.2N,
13.2O Ann Ronan Picture Library 8.5I, 9.4Q Royal College of Surgeons
(bottom box p. 75), cover, 10.1A Science Photo Library 12.1G Ronald
Sheridan/Ancient Art and Architecture Collection 3E, 4.2D Paul Shuter
p.35 Topham Picture Library 12.3M University of Bradford,
Department of Archaeological Sciences, Calvin Wells Collection 1.2D
Wellcome Institute Library 2.5I, 4.2C, 7.3C, 7.6H, 12.1F, 12.2J, 12.4Z,
13.1C, 13,2E, 13.3(1) Werner Forman Archive 7.5G, 12.4X
West Stowe Country Park 6D Zentrale Farbbild Agentur 9.1B

Thanks are also due to *Health Which?* December 1992, published by
Consumers' Association, 2 Marylebone Rd, London NW1 4DF for the
chart on page 120.

Details of written sources

In some sources the wording or sentence structure has been simplified
to ensure that the source is accessible.

Paul Addison, 'A New Jerusalem', in *Britain 1918-51*, Heinemann
Educational, 1994: 13.2M
Paul Addison, *Now the War is Over*, Cape, 1985: 13.2P, 13.2R
Michael Alexander, *Earliest English Poems*, Penguin, 1966: 6A
W.J. Bishop, *Early History of Surgery*, 1960: 7.4E
Marie Boas, *The Scientific Renaissance 1450-1630*, Penguin, 1972: 9.2C
Derrick Boxley, *Jenner and Smallpox Vaccine*, Heinemann, 1981:
11.1E, 11.1F
R.A. Browne, *British Latin Selections, AD 500-1400*, Blackwell, 1954: 8.7Y
J. Chadwick, W.N. Mann, I. M. Ionie & E.T. Withington, *Hippocratic
Writings*, Penguin, 1983: 4.3G, 4.8(2)
R. J. Cootes, *The Welfare State*, Longman, 1970: 13.2Q
Nancy Dunn & Dr Jenny Sutcliffe, *A History of Medicine From Prehistory
to the Year 200*, Simon and Schuster, 1992: 12.1A
M. W. Flynn (ed.), *A Report of the Sanitary Conditions of the Labouring
Population of Great Britain*, Edinburgh University Press, 1965:
13.1F, 13.1H
GLC, *A History of the Black Presence in London*, GLC, 1986: 12.4W
H. L. Gordon, *Sir James Young Simpson and Chloroform*, 1897: 12.1E
W. A. Greenhill (trans.), *A Treatise on the Smallpox and Measles by Rhazes*,
Sydenham Society, 1848: 7.3D
Alastair McIntosh Gray, *Medical Care and Public Health: 1780 to the Present
Day*, OUP, 1990: 11.5Q, 11.5R
Douglas Guthrie, *A History of Medicine*, Nelson, 1945: 8.5J
Knut Haeger, *The Illustrated History of Surgery*, Harold Starke, 1988: 12.1D
W. O. Hassall, *They Saw it Happen 55BC-1485*, Blackwell, 1956: 6B
Nigel Kelly, *Medieval Realms*, Heinemann Educational, 1993: 8.1A
Geoffrey Keynes, *The Apologie and Treatise of Ambrose Paré*, Falcon
Educational Books, 1951: 9.3J, 9.3K, 9.3L, 9.3M
Hugh Lloyd Jones, *The Greek World*, Penguin, 1965: 5.6(1)
W.H.S. Jones, *Pliny's Natural History*, Heinemann, 1923: 5.6(2)
M. V. Lyons, *Medicine in the Medieval World*, Macmillan, 1984: 8.2B,
8.2C, 8.5K
R. H. Major, *Classic Descriptions of Disease*, Charles S. Thompson Inc.,
1945: 8.7P, 8.7S, 8.7V, 8.7W
V. Nutton, 'A Social History of Graeco-Roman Medicine', in *Medicine in
Society* (ed A. Wear) CUP, 1994: 5.2B
E.D. Phillips, *Greek Medicine*, Thames and Hudson, 1975: 4.2E, 4.5H,
4.5J, 4.5(1)
Colin Platt, *The English Medieval Town*, Granada, 1979: 8.6N
Dodie Poynter, *History at Source: Medicine 300-1929*, Evans Bros., 1971:
11.5(4)
Robert Reid, *Microbes and Men*, BBC, 1974: 11.6 (2 & 3), 12.2I
Philip Rhodes, *An Outline of the History of Medicine*, 1985: 12.4V
J. D. de C. M. Saunders & Charles D. O'Malley, *The Illustrations for the
Works of Andreas Vesalius*, World Publishing, 1950, 9.2D
SCHP, *Medicine Through Time: A Study in Development*, Book 1, Holmes
McDougal, 1976: 8.7P, 8.7Q, 8.7R
SCHP, *Medicine Through Time: A Study in Development*, Book 3, Holmes
McDougal, 1976: 811.4P, 13.1I
Joe Scott, *Medicine Through Time*, Holmes McDougal, 1987: 11.1G
Dr Thomas Shapter, *A History of the Cholera in Exeter in 1832*, 1841: 13.1D
Richard Shyrock, *The Development of Modern Medicine*, 1948: 12.6(2)
Charles Singer & E.A. Underwood, *A Short History of Medicine*, Oxford
1962: 4.7M
Charles Singer, *Galen On Anatomical Procedures*, London 1956: 5.5K
G. Sweetman, *A History of Wincanton*, 1903: 11.1D
Hugh Thomas, *Spain*, 1964: 7.2A
Lynn Thorndike, *Michael Scot*, Nelson, 1965: 8.3E
R. Vallery-Radot, *Life of Pasteur*, London, 1911: 11.2H
J. J. Walsh, *Medieval Medicine*, 1920: 6C
Leo M. Zimmermann & Ilza Veith, *Great Ideas in the History of Surgery*,
1961: 12.2K

CONTENTS

PREHISTORIC MEDICINE

1.1 What was the prehistoric period?

For historians, a prehistoric society is one without writing. Although the prehistoric period does not have a definitive starting point and finishing point, historians usually say it started about 500,000 years ago. All of the evidence we are studying, however, comes from the last 20,000 years.

Prehistoric people lived throughout the world. Not all peoples in the world left the prehistoric period at the same time. Once writing developed in a society, that society was no longer prehistoric. So Britain was still prehistoric long after Egypt and the Middle East, where writing developed much earlier.

The earliest prehistoric peoples had the following features in common.

- They were nomads.
- They were hunter gatherers – so they got all their food without farming.
- They lived in small groups without complicated political arrangements. There were no separate countries.
- They had a very simple level of technology – spears, bows and arrows, axes, knives and scrapers were their main tools. All of these were made from wood, bone and stone.
- They had no system of writing.

Over thousands of years things changed slowly. The most important changes were the development of farming (which meant people stayed in one place) and metal tools.

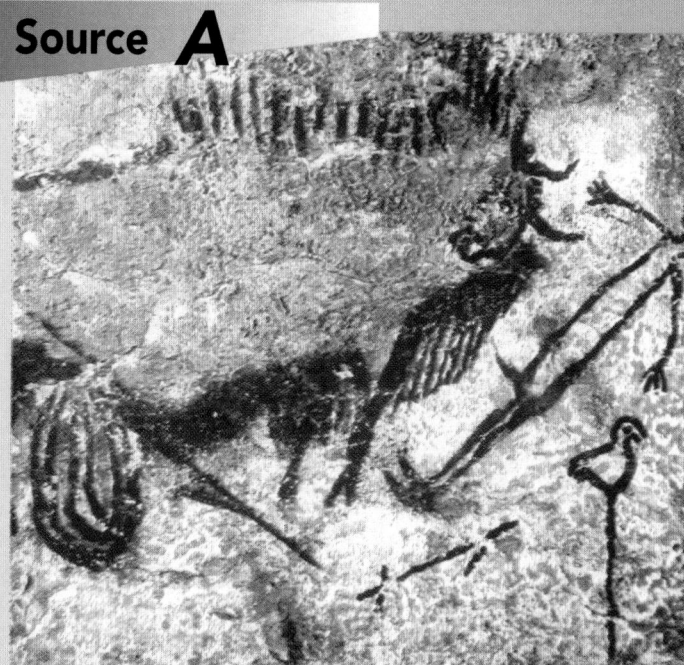

▲ A cave painting made by prehistoric people in France about 15,000 years ago.

QUESTIONS

1 Look at each of the common features of early prehistoric peoples listed on this page.

a Explain the feature.

b How do you think it might have affected the medicine they used, and our ability to find out about their medicine?

Old Stone Age				New Stone Age		Bronze Age	Iron Age
18000 BC	15000 BC	12000 BC	9000 BC	6000 BC	3000 BC	0	AD 2000

Cave paintings in France
Sources A and C

▲ The Stone Age (in most of Europe and the Middle East).

1.2 Prehistoric medicine

We can tell that prehistoric people suffered injury and disease. Their bones show us this. What we do not know, however, is if, or how, they treated themselves.

Source B

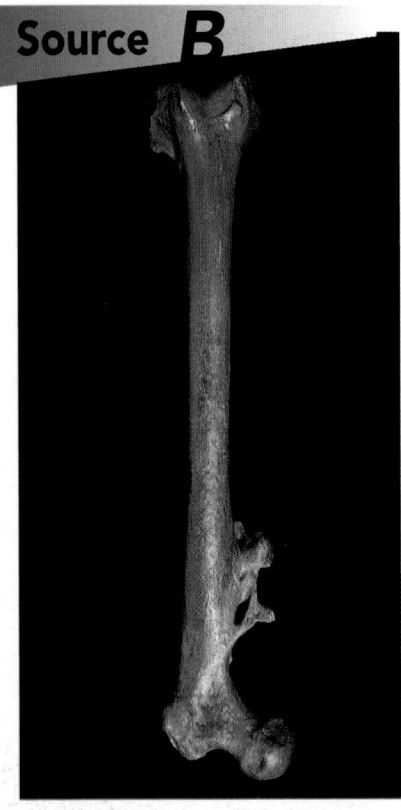

▲ The thigh bone of a prehistoric person. You can clearly see a large growth on the bone.

Source C

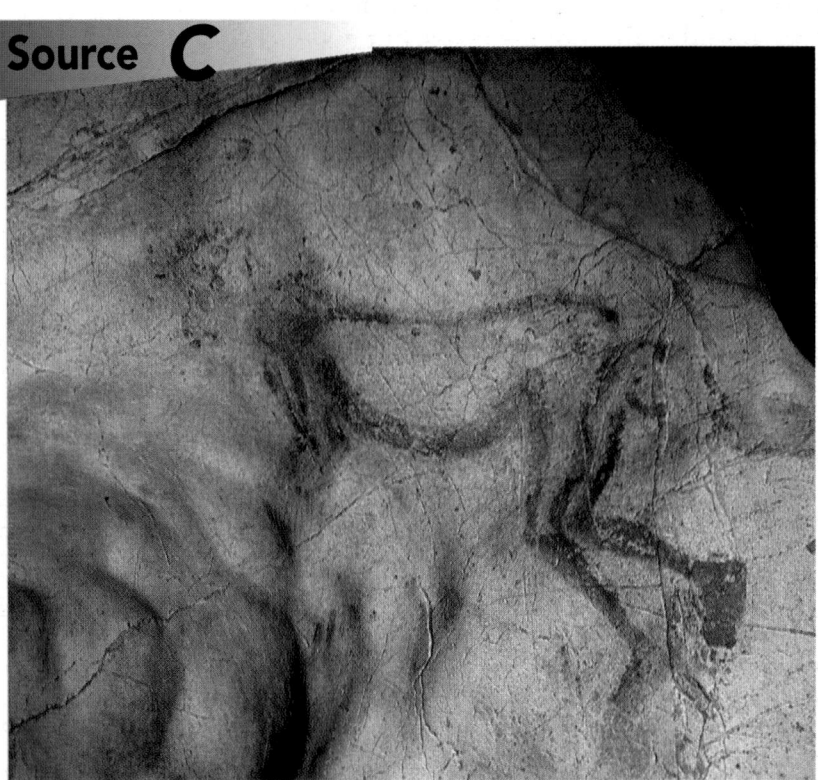

▲ A cave painting made by prehistoric people in France about 15,000 years ago. We cannot be sure exactly what this painting shows, but many other prehistoric paintings show a man with antlers like this one, often standing in a circle with twelve other men.

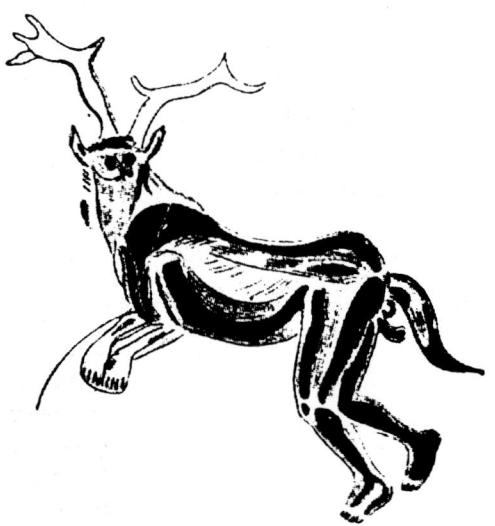

▶ This modern drawing of the cave painting in Source C shows the outline of a man with antlers, possibly wearing a mask, more clearly.

Trephined skulls have been found in almost every part of the world where prehistoric people lived. Trephining is when a hole is cut in a person's skull while they are still alive. Both men's and women's skulls have been found with trephine holes, but never a child's skull. They are found in burial sites with the complete body of the person. Often the piece of bone that was cut out of the skull was found in the grave with the body. Often this piece of skull had one or two holes made in it, perhaps so it could have been threaded on a thong and worn round the neck. Most of the skulls have bone growth around the hole made by the operation. This means that these persons lived on, probably for many years. Historians have to work out why this operation, which must have been both painful and dangerous, was done. These are the main theories historians have put forward since these skulls were first found in the 1860s:

Theory 1: Dr Prunieres (1865) suggested the holes were made in the skulls so they could be used as drinking vessels.

Theory 2: Professor Paul Broca (1876) suggested the operation was performed on children, and those who survived were thought to have great magic power. When the person died, the skull and the piece taken out were used as very powerful charms.

Theory 3: E. Guiard (1930) suggested trephining operations were originally performed on people who had skull injuries and, later, on people with other problems, perhaps epilepsy or very bad headaches.

Theory 4: Douglas Guthrie (1945) suggested that the operation may have been performed to let evil spirits out of the body.

QUESTIONS

1 Look at sources B–D. For each source

   a Say whether it is **definitely** evidence that prehistoric people suffered from disease.

   b Say whether it tells us anything about how prehistoric people treated disease.

2 We can be sure that some of the theories about trephining given on this page are wrong as they are contradicted by the evidence. Some of them may be right or they may not – we cannot be sure. Look at each theory in turn.

   a Describe the theory.

   b Say whether you think the theory is definitely wrong, could be right or wrong, or is definitely right.

   c Explain why the evidence of the sources supports your answer to part **b**.

Source D

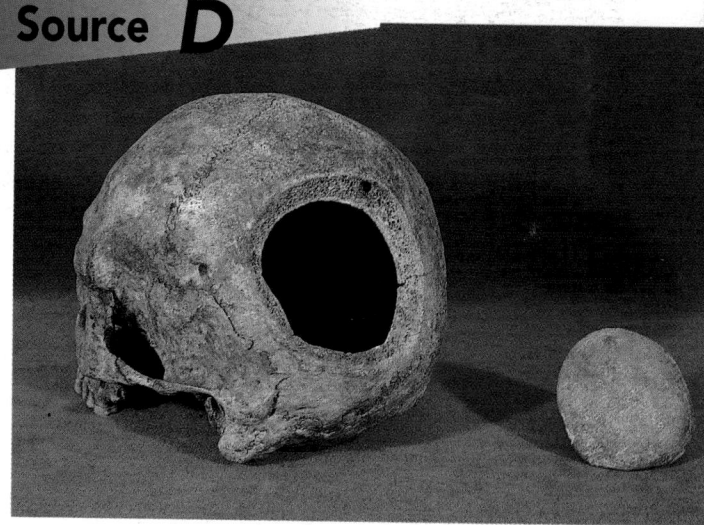

▲ A skull of a prehistoric adult found, in 1938, at Crichel Down in Dorset. The hole in the skull was cut out while the person was alive. They probably lived for many years after the operation because the bone grew a little where it was cut – rounding off the edge. The disc of bone that was cut out of the skull was buried with the person.

Historians and evidence

Historians have a real problem interpreting the evidence about prehistoric medicine. We know some facts. There was illness. Trephining operations were performed. We do not know what people thought about illness though, and we do not know why trephining operations were done. To help provide explanations, historians have looked at the medical beliefs of various groups around the world whose technology and lifestyle are similar to prehistoric people.

The Aborigines of central and southern Australia were visited by anthropologists during the late 19th and early 20th centuries. Before these visits, the Aborigines had little or no contact with the European settlers in Australia. The Aborigines lived in the harsh conditions of the Australian desert. They obtained their food by hunting and by gathering wild plants. They were nomads, moving from water hole to water hole. They had many spoken languages but no written one. In all these ways they were very similar to prehistoric people.

Aboriginal spirits

The Aborigines thought the world started in the dreamtime when the spirit ancestors lived. Many things in their world were hard to explain – why was there a stream or a water hole in one place and not another? Their answer was because the spirit ancestors had put one there. Spirits were also thought to be the cause of new life – whether human or animal. Anything which did not have an obvious physical explanation was explained as the work of spirits.

The causes of illness

This division, between things with an obvious cause and things without an obvious cause, was part of aboriginal medicine. Some problems were treated with common-sense cures:

- Broken arms were encased in clay which would set hard in the sun – very like a modern plaster cast.
- Cuts were covered with clay or animal fat and bound up with bark or animal skin.

Other problems did not have an obvious cause. Aborigines had two explanations for these. The first was that an evil spirit had entered the sick person's body. The second was that the person's own spirit had left, or been taken, from his or her body. If an enemy had captured the sick person's spirit with a pointing bone (see page 9), then the treatment was to try and find the bone, which would have the spirit stuck to it. If the illness was thought to be caused by an evil spirit in the person's body then the treatment would try to drive that spirit out. This gives us an important insight into the history of medicine. The cures people used were related to what they thought caused the disease. If the disease was thought to have a spiritual cause, then only a spiritual cure would make sense.

THE PREHISTORIC PERIOD

Historians divide the prehistoric period into a number of different eras:

Old Stone Age (Palæolithic) when people were nomadic hunter gatherers.

New Stone Age (Neolithic) when farming and living in one place became common.

Bronze Age when metal tools were first used.

Iron Age when the new metal greatly improved the tools and weapons which could be made.

There was an overlap in time between the prehistoric period and those described in the next chapters. Most of Europe was in the New Stone Age during the height of the Egyptian civilization. The Minoan civilization happened at the same time as the Bronze Age in other places, and Britain was in the Iron Age during the Greek and early Roman periods.

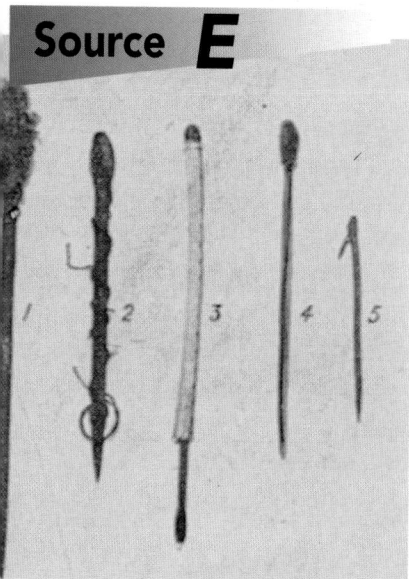

▲ Aborigine pointing bones and sticks like these had gum on the ends. They were said to control the spirits when used in special ceremonies.

Source **F**

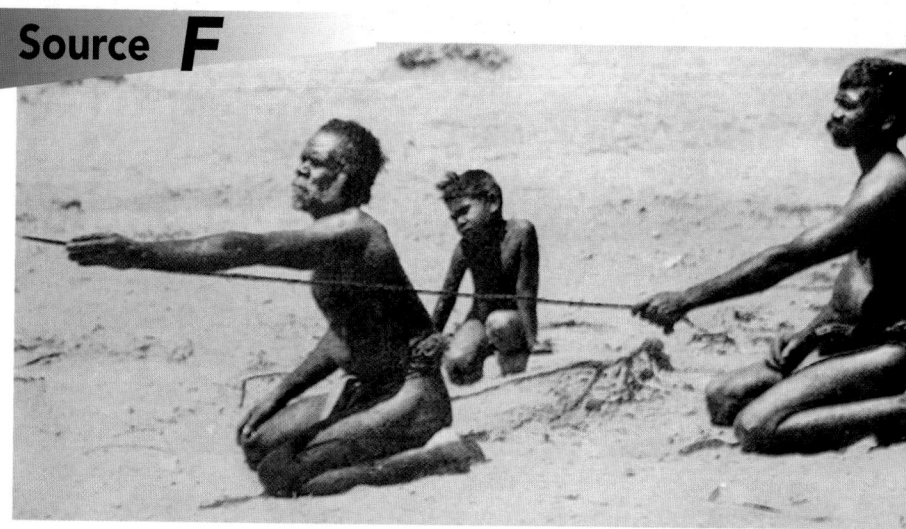

▲ These Aborigines are chanting and pointing a special 'death bone', which they believed gave them the power to kill from a distance.

QUESTIONS

1 In what ways were 19th century Aborigines like prehistoric people?

2 a Describe an Aboriginal common-sense treatment.

 b Why do you think they did not use a spirit cure for this treatment?

3 a Describe an Aboriginal spiritual treatment.

 b Why do you think they did not use a common-sense treatment for this problem?

4 Do you think Aborigines would use spiritual or common-sense treatments for the following problems?

 a A sprained wrist caused in a fall.

 b A heart attack.

 c An epileptic fit.

 d A spear wound.

Explain the reasons for your answer in each case.

1.5 Conclusions

The 19th century aboriginal way of life was very similar to what we know about the way of life of prehistoric people. The ideas of the aborigines may therefore help us understand the ideas of prehistoric people. If the aborigines used both common sense and a belief in spirits in their medicine, so might prehistoric people. The man shown in Source C (page 6) may have been a medicine man. The medicine man's (or woman's) explanation for many illnesses may have been that they were caused by evil spirits. Trephining operations may have been performed to let out evil spirits through the hole in the skull. The pieces of skull removed in the operation may have been worn as a charm to keep evil spirits away. This is the view of prehistoric medicine that historians think is most likely. However, it is only a theory. Because we have no written records from prehistoric times, we cannot be sure what people really thought.

The chart below summarizes the important information about prehistoric medicine. There is one of these charts for each chapter in the first half of the book. Completing the chart is a useful way to look back over the material you have just studied, to make sure you understand it. Correctly filled in charts will be useful for revision. Notice how many of the sections of the chart have a place for *Evidence*. Good historians can always support what they say with evidence and so should you when you take exams. Filling in these sections of the chart will give you useful practice in selecting the facts which you can use to back up answers.

The chart is split into four different sections:

Factors affecting Medicine which is explained in more detail on the right.

Causes of Disease which is concerned with what people thought caused disease at the time.

Treatments Used where you can record some of the ways in which injury and diseases were treated.

New Features where you need to think about each period in relation to the ones which went before.

Factors affecting Medicine

This section is about the factors that have influenced change and development. The most important factors are:

Science and/or Technology for example, our highly developed science and technology, with x-rays and ultrasound helps medicine because it allows doctors to discover what is happening inside the body.

War for example, plastic surgery was developed during World War Two to help air crew with new and terrible burns.

Religion for example, some religious groups today do not allow blood transfusions.

Government and the way society is organized and run; for example, the creation of the National Health Service and state funded medicine in Britain in 1948.

Communications from the development of writing to air transport; for example, modern transplants are often only possible because organs can be flown from one hospital to another.

Chance, unplanned events; for example, penicillin was first found when Alexander Fleming was checking through the remains of old and failed experiments.

Copy and complete the summary chart below.

Prehistoric Medicine					
Factors affecting Medicine		**Causes of Disease**		**New Features**	
Factor	Effect	Cause	Evidence	Feature	Evidence
1 _____	No method of writing so difficult to preserve knowledge or pass it on accurately so progress difficult.	**1** Supernatural: a) Loss of a person's spirit b) Evil spirit in the body	_____ _____	**1** Spirits thought to cause disease.	
		2 Physical: simple injuries like a broken arm or leg			
2 _____	An unstable society, large scale projects and long term planning almost impossible so progress difficult.	**Treatments Used**			**2** Medicine men or women – special people to treat the sick.	a) Aborigines b) _____
		Treatment	Illness	Evidence	
		1 _____	Cannot be sure	Skulls (Source D)	
		2 Encased in clay	_____	Aborigines	
		3 Covered with clay or animal fat and bound with bark or animal skin.	Cuts	_____	**3** Magical cures	a) _____ b) _____
3 _____	No understanding of how the body worked so progress difficult.	**4** _____	Any disease without an obvious physical cause.	Aborigines	**4** Common sense cures	Aborigines

CHAPTER 2

EGYPTIAN MEDICINE

2.1 Ancient Egypt

Life in Ancient Egypt

The Ancient Egyptian civilization lasted for about 2,600 years, from around 3000 BC to about 400 BC. Egypt was a well-organized and hierarchical society, from the pharaoh and the vizier at the top, to the peasants who worked the land at the bottom. The physical geography of the country forced people to settle along the banks of the river Nile. The Nile flooded once a year. This kept the surrounding land very fertile. Successful farming of this land left the Egyptians time for other things. They developed into a specialized society. There were priests, scribes, lawyers and doctors, as well as craftsmen like the stonemasons and painters who made the great buildings. Sons were trained by their fathers from an early age in the same job. In some professions, including medicine, a father might train his daughter to do his job if he had no sons.

The most important difference between the Egyptians and prehistoric people was that the Egyptians had developed writing. The developmant of writing affected their medicine. It meant they could write about illnesses and treatments, and so keep a record of those treatments that worked and those that did not. This enabled them to develop their treatments by trial and error.

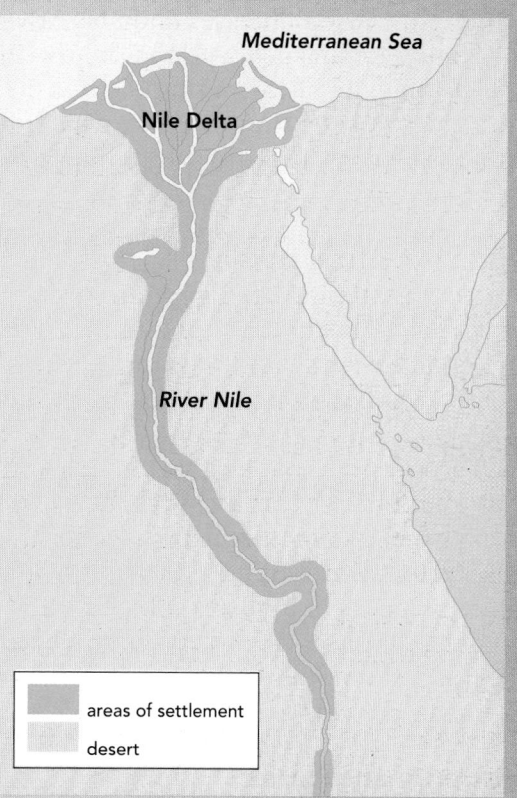

Mediterranean Sea

Nile Delta

River Nile

areas of settlement

desert

Egyptian religion

The Egyptians were very religious and believed in many gods. These gods made everything happen, from the rising of the sun to the flooding of the river Nile each year, without which the Egyptians would not have been able to grow crops. Some of these gods were thought to cause and cure disease. The goddess of war, Sekhmet, was also thought to cause and cure epidemics. Thoth is described in a medical book, the *Papyrus Ebers*, as the god who 'gives physicians the skill to cure'.

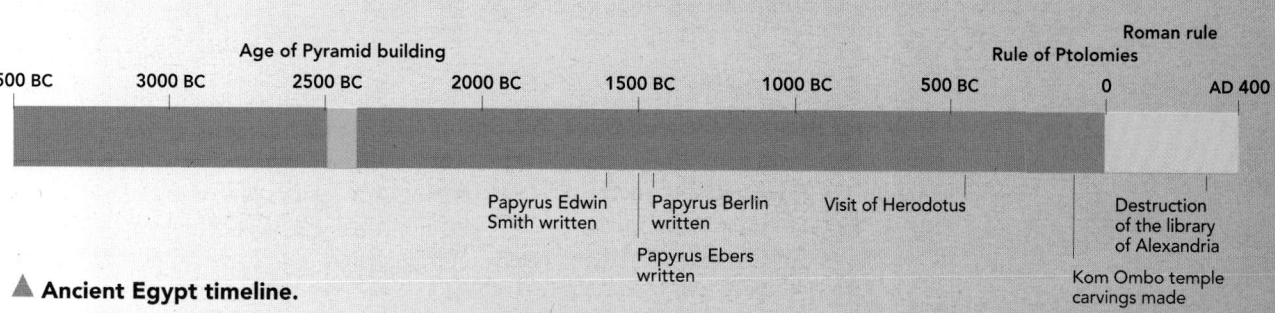

Roman rule

Rule of Ptolomies

Age of Pyramid building

| 3500 BC | 3000 BC | 2500 BC | 2000 BC | 1500 BC | 1000 BC | 500 BC | 0 | AD 400 |

Papyrus Edwin Smith written

Papyrus Berlin written

Papyrus Ebers written

Visit of Herodotus

Destruction of the library of Alexandria

Kom Ombo temple carvings made

▲ Ancient Egypt timeline.

Because the Egyptians left written records, we know what they thought caused illnesses and also how they treated them. The Egyptians believed that many diseases were caused by an evil spirit entering the body. They often wore charms to keep these spirits away. If they became ill despite the charms, they turned to magic and the gods to make them well.

Egyptian medical books

The most important early Egyptian medical books were the *Books of Thoth*. They were kept by his priests in the temple of Thoth, god of writing and wisdom. None of these books have survived but a medical book from about 1500 BC that has survived, the *Papyrus Ebers*, was probably based on them. These kind of books give very clear instructions on how to treat illness. This includes the exact words to be spoken as well as any medicine or other treatment to be given. Doctors were supposed to follow the procedure outlined precisely. If a doctor followed the procedures and the patient still died, the doctor was not blamed. If, however, the doctor did not follow the book precisely and the patient died, the doctor was executed.

Treatments and cures

The first herbal cures and drugs (made from minerals, herbs and animal parts) were probably given as part of the magical cure, not as an alternative to magic. They were intended to drive the evil spirit away, perhaps because of their smell or bitter taste. Drugs were either boiled and strained, or pounded to a fine powder. They were then mixed up and given with wine, water or beer. They were sometimes mixed into pills with dough, or mixed with honey. Chest diseases were often treated by making the patient inhale steam. Wounds and skin conditions were treated with ointments. Many of the Egyptians' drugs are still used, in a different form, in medicines today. Their record keeping shows that, if a remedy worked, they kept using it. The Egyptians' faith in these remedies would probably have been as much to do with their belief in magic as their faith in a particular drug.

Source A

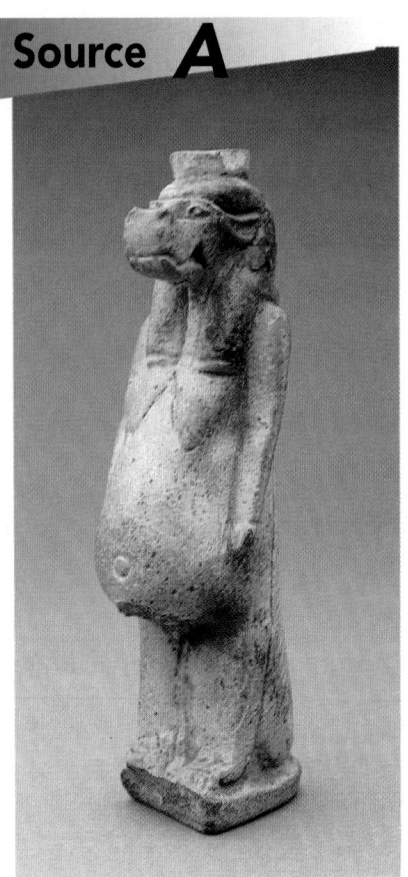

▲ An amulet of the goddess Taweret. Taweret, a pregnant hippopotamus, was the goddess of childbirth. Taweret's face is shown looking fierce to drive away evil spirits which might affect either the mother or the baby. These amulets were worn by pregnant women to keep themselves safe during pregnancy and childbirth, which, for them, was a very dangerous time.

▶ A spell from the *Papyrus Ebers*. The doctor was to chant this spell while giving the patient the medicine. The Egyptian doctor who used the papyrus had written next to the spell, 'This spell is really excellent – successful many times.' The *Papyrus Ebers* was made about 1500 BC.

Source B

Here is the great remedy. Come! You who drive evil things from my stomach and my limbs. He who drinks this shall be cured just as the gods above were cured.

QUESTIONS

1 What were the main differences between life in Ancient Egypt and prehistoric times?

2 Why are Egyptian medical books important to historians of medicine?

3 What do the *Books of Thoth* and the *Papyrus Ebers* tell us about what the Egyptians thought caused disease?

EGYPTIAN MEDICAL BOOKS

Only a few medical books have survived from Ancient Egypt. They were written on papyrus, a kind of paper made from reeds. The books we know about have been found by archaeologists. They are known by the name of the modern owner, or museum where they are kept. The *Papyrus Edwin Smith* was bought by Smith, an American egyptologist, in 1862. It was written about 1600 BC and considers wounds and the work of surgeons as well as treatments and drugs. The *Papyrus Ebers*, written about 1500 BC, contains over 700 remedies. It is named after a German egyptologist, Maurice Ebers, who acquired it in 1873. The *Papyrus Berlin*, owned by the Berlin Museum, was written about 1450 BC, and concentrates on the treatment and protection of mothers and babies.

2.3 Religion and anatomy

Anatomy is the study of the structure of the body. Knowing how the body is made up, and how it works, is an important part of medicine. The Egyptians learned some anatomy as an unintended consequence of their religious beliefs. They believed that after a person died, his or her soul left the body. After a while the soul returned to the body and the person then began an afterlife, very like the life they had led before they died. It was important, therefore, to keep dead bodies in good condition for their souls to use when they returned.

Source C

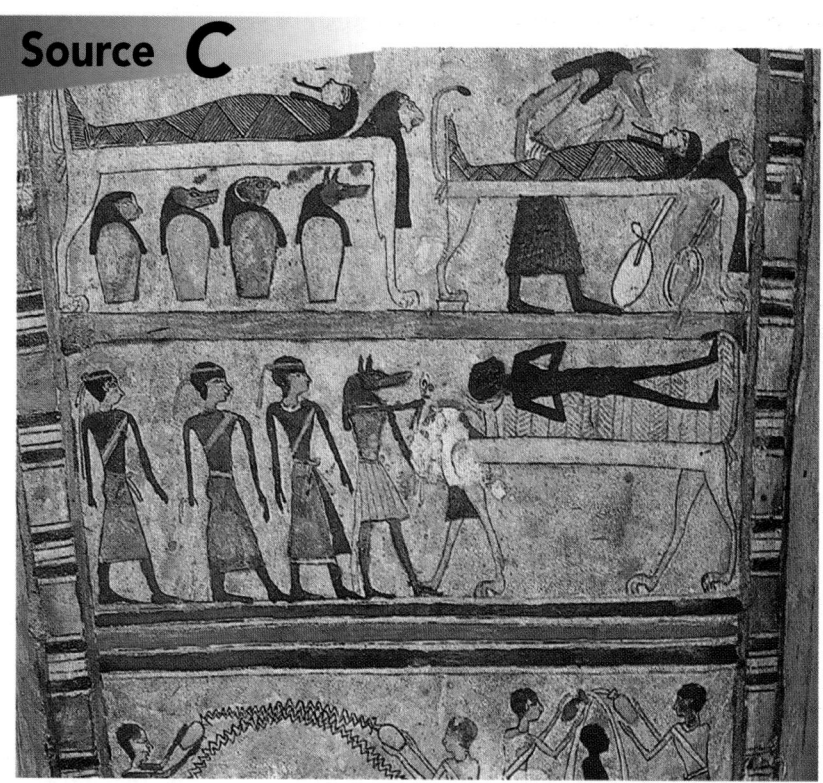

▲ Parts of the mummification process from a painted coffin from around 600 BC. The lower section shows the body (darker in colour than the living people) being washed in a natron (sodium chloride) solution. The middle section shows the body covered with natron crystals during the 40 day drying-out stage. At the top, on the left, the mummy has been placed in its tomb with the *canopic* jars underneath. They held the liver, lungs, stomach and intestines. On the right the god Anubis is attending to the mummy.

Source D

Forty-six vessels go from the heart to every limb. If a doctor, surgeon or exorcist places his hands or fingers on the back of the head, hands, stomach, arms or feet, then he hears the heart. The heart speaks out of every limb.

▲ From the *Papyrus Ebers*, about 1500 BC.

The Egyptians devoted much time to finding out ways of preserving bodies. They soaked the bodies in various liquids, including salts and bitumen. They covered them in oils and wrapped them in bandages. This process was called embalming, and the embalmed bodies were called mummies.

Embalming included cutting open the body to take out the main organs (heart, lungs, liver, spleen, brain) because they would rot. They were kept whole and stored with the mummy in canopic jars. The process of embalming gave the Egyptians a good understanding of some parts of human anatomy. Removing the major organs meant they knew where they were located inside the body. But their belief in the afterlife, which meant that they carried out the embalming in the first place, prevented them from doing any further research into the structure of the body. Because the body was needed for the afterlife it could not be further dissected.

Source E

In the best treatment, first of all they draw out the brains through the nostrils with an iron hook. When they have removed what they can in this way they flush out the remainder with drugs. Next they make a cut in the side, with an obsidian knife, through which they take out all the internal organs. They clean out the body cavity, rinsing it with palm wine and powdered spices, and then they stitch it up again. When they have done this, they cover the corpse in natron for 70 days and so mummify it. Then they wash the corpse and wrap it from head to toe in linen bandages smeared with the finest gum. Finally the relatives put it in a man-shaped wooden coffin and store it in a burial chamber, where it is propped upright against the wall. This is the most costly method of preparing the dead.

▲ A description of one of the methods of mummification from *The Histories*, a book written by Herodotus, a Greek traveller and historian who visited Egypt about 450 BC.

2.4 A natural theory of the causes of disease

The river Nile was vital to Egyptian life. Every year the river flooded. Its waters were dammed and channelled into irrigation ditches to keep the crops growing. This control of the flood waters by damming gave some doctors an alternative theory about the cause of disease. They thought the human body might be full of channels, rather like the irrigation system. Their knowledge of anatomy told them that there were many vessels inside the body through which blood and other fluids flowed. If an irrigation channel got blocked, the life giving water would not flow into the fields. Perhaps the same thing happened inside the human body? If one of the vessels became blocked would the person become ill?

This was a very different idea about the causes of disease from those held earlier.

Now the disease was believed to have a physical as well as a spiritual cause. That meant the treatment should include the physical as well. These Egyptian doctors used a variety of treatments:

- Vomiting was thought to be good for some patients. It might clear blockages in some parts of the body.
- Purges (medicines that worked as laxatives), were often used. They might clear some blockages from the stomach and bowel.
- Bleeding was also used. A doctor would deliberately cut a vein so that the patient lost a certain amount of blood. This, it was thought, might clear any blockages in the blood vessels.

These methods were not accepted by everyone, nor did doctors who used them reject spiritual explanations for disease. The treatments in the *Papyrus Ebers* show both the **natural** and the **supernatural** theories of the causes of disease.

Source F

There are two vessels in the arm. If he is ill in his arm then let him vomit by means of fish and beer and bandage his fingers with water melon until he is healed. If he is ill in the bowel the blockage must be cleared. **Colocynth**, senna, fruit of sycamore are ground together into a paste and shaped into four cakes for him to eat.

▲ Treatment from the *Papyrus Ebers*, about 1500 BC.

2.5 Surgery

Surgery, like all crafts in Egypt, was passed on from father to son (or sometimes daughter). The *Papyrus Edwin Smith*, written in about 1600 BC, describes some simple surgical procedures, including treating dislocated arms and legs. None of the existing written records discuss major operations nor do the mummies that have so far been examined show any signs of major surgery.

On the other hand, as we have seen, the Egyptians had a reasonable grasp of human anatomy. The written evidence shows that they performed minor surgery, like the removal of cysts and tumours. Because so much surgery was done, it was likely that it was one of the medical skills in which people specialized. These minor operations probably had quite a good recovery rate, because the wounds that were left after operating were treated with willow. We now know that willow leaves and bark produce a form of antiseptic, which would have protected the wound against infection.

Source G

If you examine a man with a dislocation of his jaw where his mouth is open and he cannot close it, you should put your two thumbs on the ends of the two rami of the mandible [lower jawbone] inside the mouth. Put your fingers under his chin and make them fall back into the correct position.

▲ From the *Papyrus Edwin Smith*, about 1600 BC.

Source H

When you come across a swelling of the flesh in any part of the body of the patient and your patient is clammy and the swelling comes and goes under your finger unless the finger is still, then you must say to your patient, 'It is a tumour of the flesh. I will treat the disease. I will try to heal it with fire since **cautery** heals.' When you come across a swelling that has attacked a vessel, then it has formed a tumour in the body. If, when you examine it with your fingers, it is like a hard stone, then you should say, 'It is a tumour of the vessels. I shall treat the disease with a knife.'

▲ From the *Papyrus Ebers*, about 1500 BC.

Source I

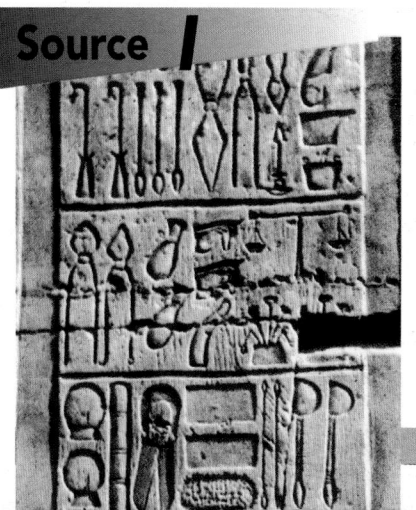

◀ Egyptian surgical instruments carved in the temple of Kom Ombo in around 100 BC. They include probes, saws, forceps, flasks, scalpels, scissors and even plants (presumably medicinal herbs to put on the wound after surgery to help it heal). Surgical instruments were mostly made from bronze, although the Egyptians used flint knives for circumcision, which had both religious and ceremonial importance.

The Egyptians believed in keeping clean. It seems that their concern with cleanliness was more to do with religion and comfort than with health. The fact that priests washed more often than other people suggests a religious connection for their washing practices. Their development of mosquito nets was more to do with comfort than the knowledge of the illnesses that mosquitoes can carry. But, whatever their reasons, their attitude to cleanliness helped them to keep healthy. Shaven heads were normal, for both men and women. Clothes were changed regularly.

Despite their sophisticated water drainage system for growing crops the Egyptians do not seem to have developed a drainage system for their toilets. Only well-off people had bathrooms and the baths were just shallow troughs with a drainage pipe leading to a large jar. Toilets were more common, but these were just stone seats over a large removable jar. Perhaps this shows that water was too valuable to be wasted in deep baths or used for sluicing away sewage, which could be carried to the fields by slaves and used as manure.

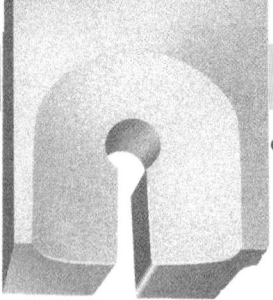

▲ An artist's reconstruction of an Egyptian toilet seat made of limestone.

Source J

The Egyptians drink from cups of bronze which they clean daily – everyone, without exception. They wear linen clothes which they make a special point of continually washing. Their priests shave their whole bodies every third day, to guard against lice, or anything else equally unpleasant while they do their religious duties. Twice a day and every night these priests wash in cold water.

▲ From *The Histories* by the Greek historian Herodotus, about 450 BC.

QUESTIONS

Copy the following statements about Egyptian medicine and underline them. Underneath each statement:

a Give some evidence to support it and explain why the evidence supports it.

b Explain whether it is a new or an old idea in the history of medicine.

1 Where there was no obvious physical cause for disease some Egyptian doctors thought disease was caused by spirits and gods.

2 Egyptian doctors knew something about anatomy. They were aware of the heart, lungs, and brain.

3 Egyptian doctors used treatments based on herbs, plants and animal parts.

4 Some Egyptian doctors thought the body was like the river Nile with channels running through it. If the channels got blocked, a person would become ill.

5 Many Egyptians thought the best way to stay healthy was to scare away the evil spirits that might cause disease, so they wore charms to help them do this.

6 Egyptians were very concerned about their personal hygiene and this helped protect their health.

7 Some Egyptian doctors gave their patients careful physical examinations.

8 Egyptian doctors treated wounds, dislocations, and tumours.

2.7 Exercise

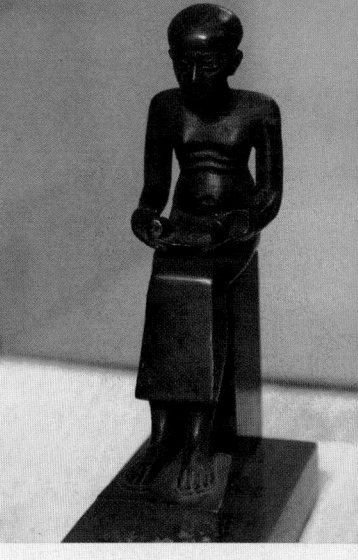

Study the sources below and then answer the questions.

Source 1

EXAMINATION
If you examine a man whose nose is disfigured – part being squashed in, while the other part is swollen and both his nostrils are bleeding.

DIAGNOSIS
Then you should say, 'You have a broken nose and this is something I can treat.'

TREATMENT
You should clean his nose with two plugs of linen and then insert two plugs soaked in grease in his nostrils. You should make him rest until his swelling has gone down, you should bandage his nose with stiff rolls of linen and treat him with lint every day until he recovers.

▲ From the *Papyrus Edwin Smith*, written in about 1600 BC.

Source 2

These words are to be spoken over the sick person: 'Oh spirit, male or female, who lurks hidden in my flesh and my limbs, get out of my flesh! Get out of my limbs!'

▲ From the *Papyrus Berlin*, written in about 1450 BC.

Source 3

▶ Imhotep, Vizier to the Pharaoh Zoser, about 2630 BC. Imhotep may have been Zoser's doctor as well. He is probably the earliest doctor whose name we know. He was later worshipped by the Egyptians as a god of healing.

Use the sources and your knowledge of Egyptian medicine to answer the questions.

1 How does Source 1 show different ideas about medicine from Sources 2 and 3?

2 Do you think an Egyptian would have been surprised that a doctor might use two different types of treatment: **natural** and **supernatural**?

3 Why was writing important in the development of medicine in Egypt?

4 Why are Egyptian medical books so important in the history of medicine?

Copy and complete the summary chart below.

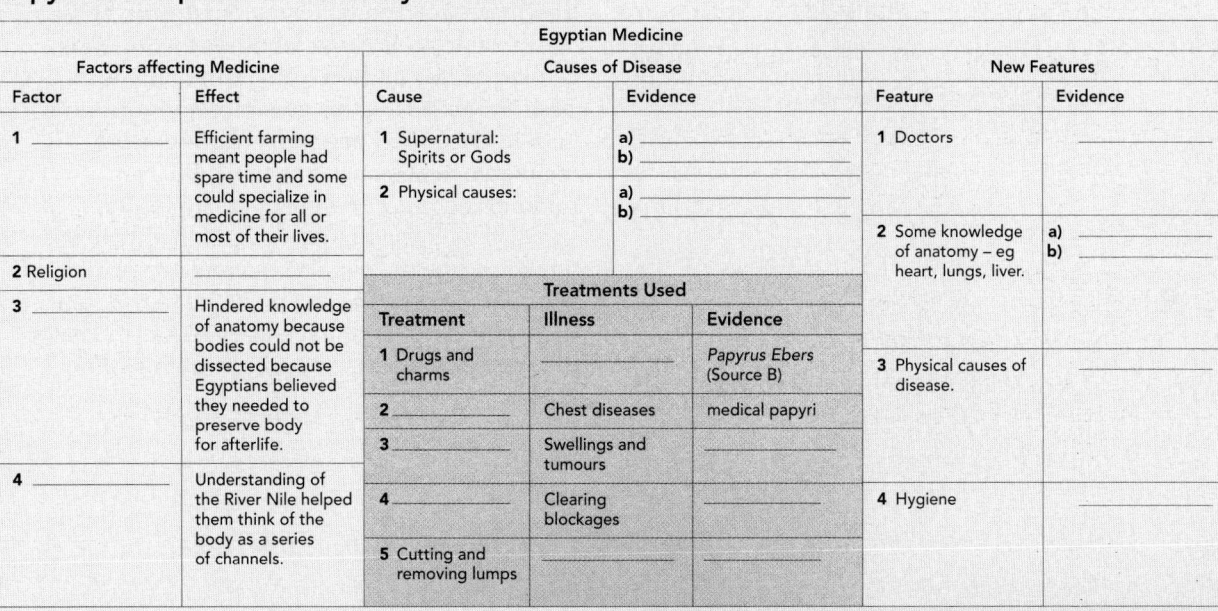

Egyptian Medicine						
Factors affecting Medicine		**Causes of Disease**			**New Features**	
Factor	Effect	Cause	Evidence		Feature	Evidence
1 _____	Efficient farming meant people had spare time and some could specialize in medicine for all or most of their lives.	1 Supernatural: Spirits or Gods	a) _____ b) _____		1 Doctors	_____
		2 Physical causes:	a) _____ b) _____			
2 Religion	_____				2 Some knowledge of anatomy – eg heart, lungs, liver.	a) _____ b) _____
3 _____	Hindered knowledge of anatomy because bodies could not be dissected because Egyptians believed they needed to preserve body for afterlife.	**Treatments Used**				
		Treatment	Illness	Evidence	3 Physical causes of disease.	_____
		1 Drugs and charms	_____	*Papyrus Ebers* (Source B)		
		2 _____	Chest diseases	medical papyri		
		3 _____	Swellings and tumours	_____		
4 _____	Understanding of the River Nile helped them think of the body as a series of channels.	4 _____	Clearing blockages	_____	4 Hygiene	_____
		5 Cutting and removing lumps	_____	_____		

CHAPTER 3

MINOAN CRETE

3.1 Who were the Minoans?

The Minoan people lived in Crete. Their civilization flourished from about 2000 BC until finally collapsing around 1380 BC. We know about the Minoan civilization because of the work of archaeologists who began excavating Minoan sites in about 1900. Previously the Minoans were known of only through legends and some references in the writings of ancient Greek authors. What the archaeologists found shows us that the Minoans had developed a civilized way of life. They were good sailors and traded widely with other Mediterranean peoples, including the Egyptians.

▼ One of the stone drains at the Minoan palace of Knossos which carried water away from the living quarters.

Source A

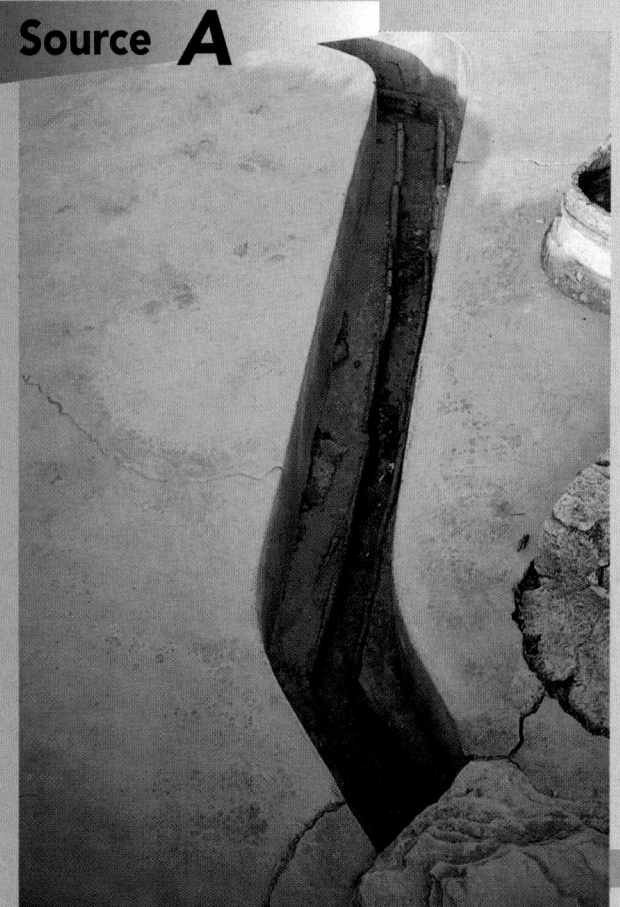

Minoan hygiene

Excavations at Knossos and other Minoan palaces show that the Minoan people developed an elaborate system of water supply and drainage. Ensuring a water supply in the dry summers of Crete must always have been a problem. In Knossos they built water tanks lined with water-resistant plaster. There were also drains covered with stone slabs to carry away sewage. Rain water was led down shafts to flush away the sewage from lavatories. Other lavatories had holes in the floor where the user or a servant could pour water from a jug to flush away the sewage. Thus the lavatories could be used even in the dry summertime.

SIR ARTHUR EVANS

The Minoan palace of Knossos was excavated by Sir Arthur Evans. After finding stones which were inscribed with a form of writing, (that has never been fully understood), he was determined to find out whether the legends of King Minos and the Labyrinth had any basis in fact. Using his own money, he bought land in Crete and began a programme of archaeological excavations in 1900. He restored some of the buildings he found, sometimes basing large wall paintings on just a few fragments. He also gave the rooms in the palace names based on what he thought their purpose might have been. Later evidence has not always supported his theories.

The Minoans also installed systems of pipes which may have been used to bring in water from a distance. It is possible that these pipes were carried across valleys by aqueducts, now long vanished. Rain water was collected by stone drains that had tanks to allow the sediment to settle before the water went into the cisterns.

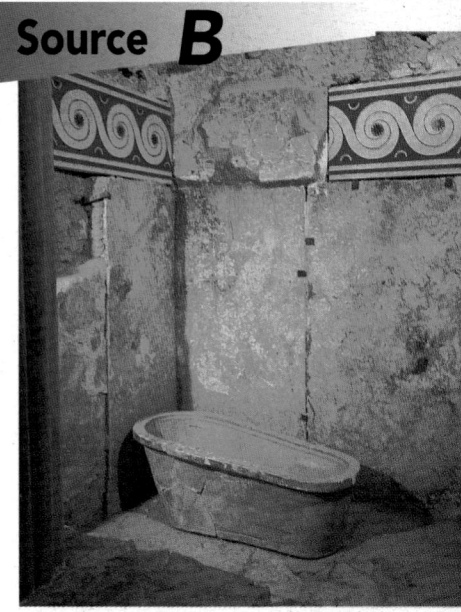

▲ The Queen's bathroom and bath in the Queen's apartments at Knossos.

3.2 The legacy of the Minoans

Historians are still arguing about the reasons why the Minoan palaces were destroyed. Some blame natural disasters like the volcanic explosion of the nearby island of Thera, that was accompanied by tidal waves and violent earth tremors. Others argue that invading Mycenaean Greeks burnt down the palaces and drove the people from the cities. What is certain is that Knossos and the other palaces were consumed by fire. The ruins remained hidden for over 3,000 years.

Thus the problems of water supply and sewage disposal that Minoan engineers had solved had to be tackled afresh by civilizations that followed. It was not until the time of the Romans that the same level of skill is found. Chance events, whether they were natural disasters or invasions of Greeks from the mainland, meant that their knowledge was lost.

QUESTIONS

1 What evidence is there that the Minoans had made advances in public health?

2 What part did the Minoans play in the development of medicine through time?

3 How does the destruction of the Minoan civilization show the effect of chance in the history of medicine?

CHANCE

We usually think of things happening for a reason. In History that reason is often to do with a person or people deciding they want something and then acting in a way that tries to make that thing happen. However many changes come about, or do not come about, because of **chance**. This means something that is unplanned, but which turns out to have a significant effect. The disappearance of the Minoan civilization is a good example. The Minoans had solved some problems of water supply and drainage which, because of the destruction of Minoan Crete, had to be solved again later. If Minoan Crete had survived this knowledge would have spread through the Greek civilization to Rome. This did not happen because of a deliberate attempt to slow down the development of medicine – it happened by chance.

ANCIENT GREECE

4.1 Greece 1000 BC – 300 BC

In the ancient world Greece was an area not a country. The people we call the Greeks lived not only in modern Greece and the Greek islands, but also in cities built on the shores of the Mediterranean, in modern Albania, Turkey, Italy, Spain and Africa. From about 1000 BC the Greeks were beginning to build cities in mainland Greece. By about 750 BC these cities had developed into independent states. Each city ruled over the surrounding countryside. The cities began to colonize by building trading settlements around the shores of the Mediterranean.

The Greeks shared a language and belief in the same gods. The early Greeks explained many of the mysteries of nature by the actions of their gods.

● The changes in the seasons were explained by the myth of Demeter and Persephone. Persephone was Demeter's daughter. For six months of every year she was forced to live in Hades – the world of the dead. This made Demeter so angry that, during this time, she would not allow plants to grow. Every spring, however, Persephone was released from Hades and Demeter, happy again, allowed the plants to grow.

● Volcanoes were caused by Hephaestos, the god of fire. He was a blacksmith and the Greeks believed that the smoke and flames from a volcano were created by Hephaestos while he worked at his forge.

◀ **The Greek world, c 450 BC.**

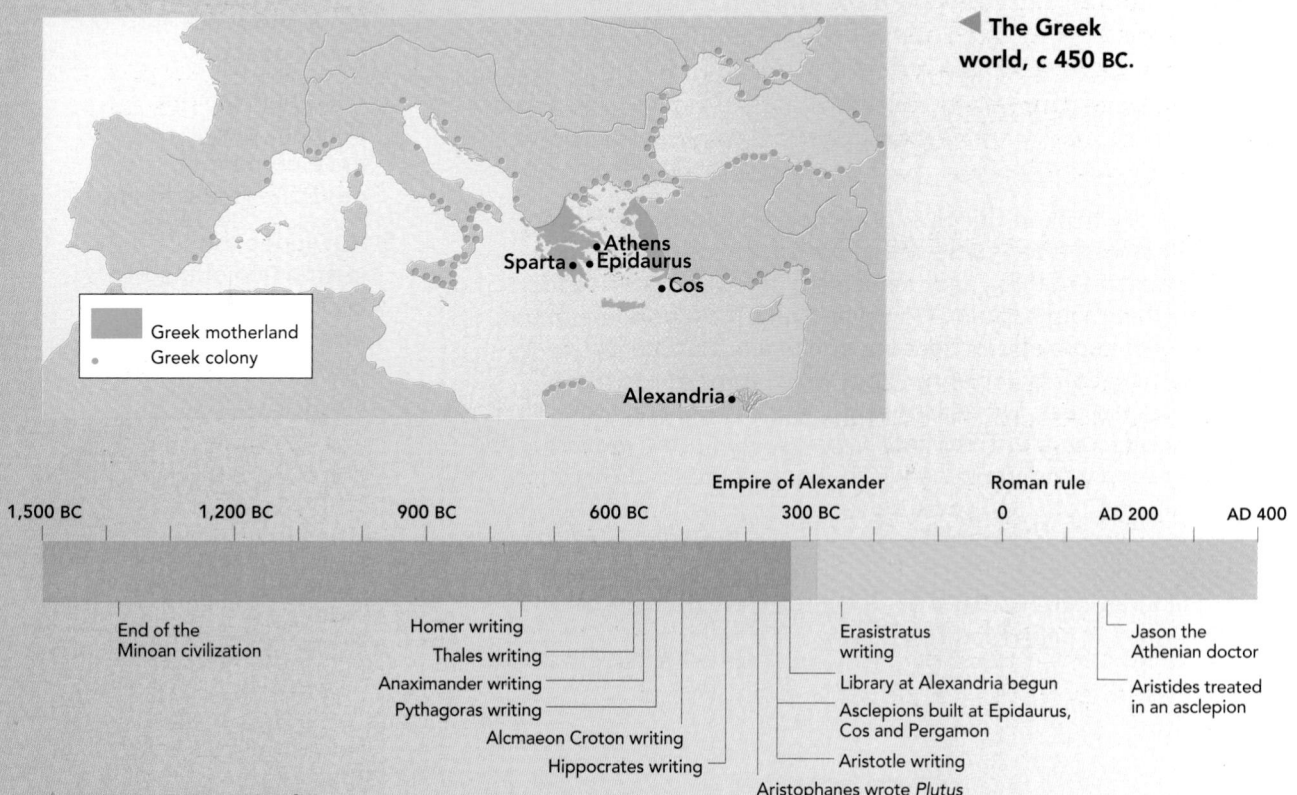

Greek motherland
Greek colony

Sparta • • Epidaurus
• Athens
• Cos

Alexandria •

Empire of Alexander   Roman rule

1,500 BC	1,200 BC	900 BC	600 BC	300 BC	0	AD 200	AD 400

End of the
Minoan civilization

Homer writing

Thales writing

Anaximander writing

Pythagoras writing

Alcmaeon Croton writing

Hippocrates writing

Aristophanes wrote *Plutus*

Aristotle writing

Asclepions built at Epidaurus, Cos and Pergamon

Library at Alexandria begun

Erasistratus writing

Jason the Athenian doctor

Aristides treated in an asclepion

▲ **Ancient Greece timeline.**

The Greek world around 450 BC

Greek civilization was at its height between 600 BC and 300 BC. The individual city states developed and became more powerful. While they were all different, they each had a leisured upper class or classes who had plenty of time to spend on their interests. Science, philosophy and mathematics were important to many Greeks. They replaced the old supernatural explanations for events with new **rational** ones produced by thinkers called philosophers. One of these, Thales of Miletus, predicted an eclipse of the sun in 585 BC because he understood some of the motions of the sun, moon and planets. He also thought water was the basis of all life. In about 560 BC Anaximander developed this theory, suggesting all things were made of four elements, earth, fire, air and water. Pythagoras, who died about 500 BC, was fascinated by mathematics. He put forward the idea that life was concerned with the balance between opposites.

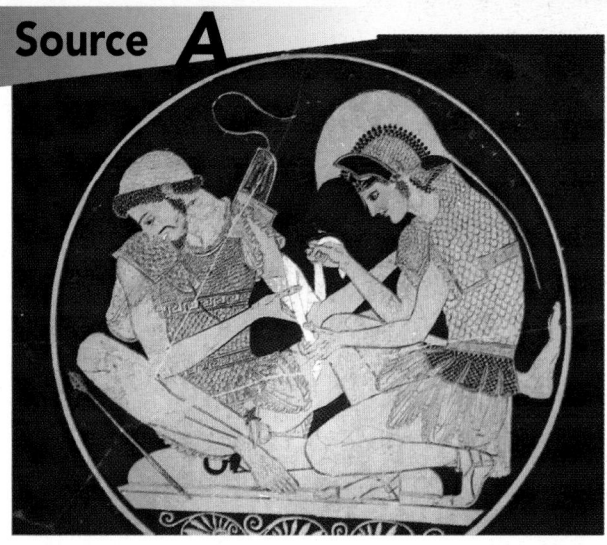

▲ A hero from the siege of Troy treats his wounded friend. This painting is from a decorated cup.

CHANGE AND DEVELOPMENT

A **change** is a completely new idea.

A **development** is when something is based on what went before it – it has *developed* from a previous idea.

Medicine developed too. Our first knowledge of Greek medicine comes from the poems of Homer. Historians believe these poems were written about 750 BC, and based on earlier poems that had been passed down by word of mouth. They tell of the siege of Troy, and of the soldiers who fought in that war. Doctors are described giving common-sense treatment to the wounds suffered by the warriors.

Two different medical traditions developed. One was the rational tradition which we associate with Hippocrates. Hippocrates was born about 460 BC and the medical books associated with him were written from about 430 BC onwards. The other was a supernatural tradition, associated with the cult of the god Asclepios. Asclepios' sons were said to have fought in the siege of Troy and stories about him were common in Homer's time. However the real growth of the cult of Asclepios came much later and the great temples that were the home of the cult were built after 400 BC. It is important to keep these dates in mind. What happened in Greece was not that a more primitive supernatural system of medicine was replaced by a more advanced natural or rational medicine. Both developed and flourished at the same time.

QUESTIONS

1 Was it possible for the Greeks to have had any contact with Egypt?

2 a Describe a change in ideas in the Greek period.

   b Describe a development in ideas in the Greek period.

   c Was Hippocratic medicine a development from the work of the philosophers?

   d Was Hippocratic medicine a development from the supernatural medicine of the cult of Asclepios?

Asclepios was the Greek god of healing. The temples built for his worship were used for treating the sick. They were called Asclepions. The cult of Asclepios became more important during the 5th century BC and the three most important Asclepions, in Epidaurus, Pergamum, and Cos, were all built or rebuilt around 350 BC.

As you can see from Source C, the Asclepions were large and complicated sites. People who were ill would go to an Asclepion, spend at least one night there, praying to Asclepios and being treated. When a sick person arrived at an Asclepion they would usually go through the following processes.

- Make an offering or sacrifice to the god.
- Bathe in the sea to cleanse and purify themselves.
- Sleep for at least one night in the *abaton*, a long thin building open to the air on each side.
- While sleeping in the abaton the patients expected to be visited by the god. Some had dreams. Others were probably treated by the priests. The snake was Asclepios' sacred animal; he is usually seen holding a staff with a snake wound round it in Greek carvings. The priests used snakes as part of the treatment in the abaton. Ointments were often rubbed into the part of the body where symptoms occurred. Sometimes the snakes licked the sick part as well.

The patient was supposed to wake up cured the next morning. Sometimes they did. Other times they did not. One of our most important sources about what happened in an Asclepion is an account written by Aristides, a philosopher from Athens, about his treatment in AD 150. Aristides had spent years visiting different Asclepions. We also have the story of a visit in a comic play, *Plutus* by Aristophanes, a Greek playwright, who died in 388 BC.

▶ **A model of the Asclepion at Epidaurus.**

Source B

First we had to bathe Plutus in the sea. Then we entered the temple where we placed our offerings to the gods on the altar. There were many sick people present, with many kinds of illnesses. Soon the temple priest put out the light and told us all to go to sleep and not to speak, no matter what noises we heard. The god sat down by Plutus. First he wiped the patient's head, then with a cloth of clean linen he wiped Plutus' eyelids a number of times. Next Panacea [*the god's daughter*] covered his face and head with a scarlet drape. The god whistled and two huge snakes appeared. They crept under the cloth and licked his eyelids. Then Plutus sat up and could see again, but the god, his helpers and the serpents had vanished.

▲ **From *Plutus*, a play written by Aristophanes. Plutus had gone to the Asclepion to be cured of blindness.**

Source C

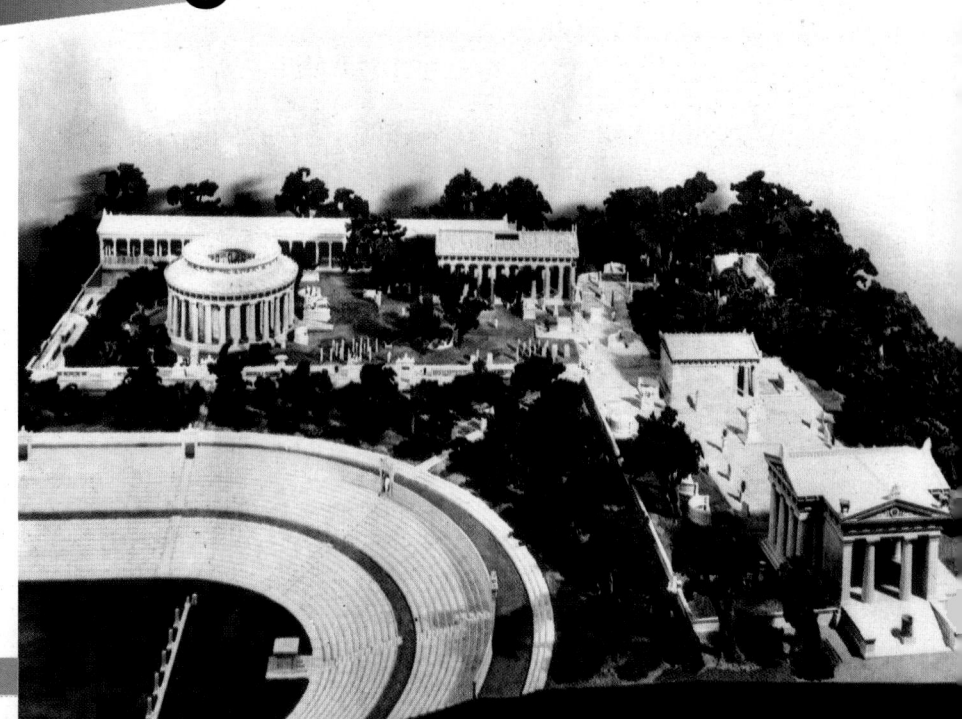

The cult of Asclepios flourished until the end of the Roman period (about AD 400). The practice of taking sick people to a religious site, in the hope they would be cured, lasted even longer. This is what happened in many medieval pilgrimages. Until the middle of the 20th century, in some Greek islands, and in parts of southern Italy and Sicily, sick people spent the night in church hoping to be cured. Cures were regularly reported. This is an example of continuity (an idea or practice that stays the same for a long time). While studying the history of medicine we tend to concentrate on change, but continuity is an important part of the overall picture.

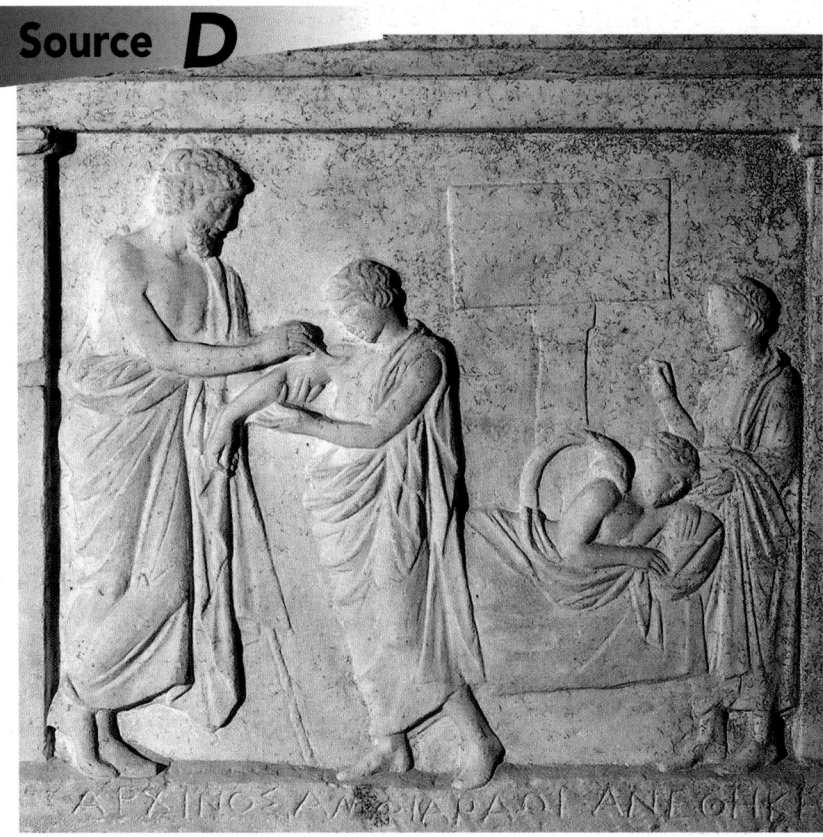

▲ A carving showing Asclepios treating a boy called Archinos, which was made about 350 BC.

Source **E**

- Ambrosia of Athens became blind in one eye. She had laughed at being told of cures to the lame and the blind. But she dreamed that Asclepios was standing beside her, saying he would cure her if she would dedicate a silver pig as a memorial to her ignorance. He seemed to cut into her diseased eyeball and pour in medicine. When she woke in the morning she was cured.

- Euhippus had had a spear point fixed in his jaw for six years. As he was sleeping in the temple Asclepios pulled out the spear point and gave it to him. When day came he left, cured and holding the spear point.

- A man had his toe healed by a serpent. While he slept a snake crawled out of the shrine and licked his diseased toe. He woke cured, saying he had dreamed that a beautiful young man had put a drug on his toe.

▲ A small selection from the stone inscriptions set into a wall of the Asclepion at Epidaurus. Such inscriptions, called *Iamata* record cures said to have happened in the temple. Archaeologists have found and translated many such inscriptions.

QUESTIONS

1 'Asclepions were both popular and successful.'

   What evidence can you find to support this statement?

2 We have a number of sources of evidence about the cult of Asclepios. Study each source in turn and answer the following questions.

   a When it was made?

   b How useful is it (what does it tell us)?

   c How reliable is it (should we believe it)?

The work of two earlier philosophers was important to Hippocrates. Pythagoras (about 580–500 BC) taught that a healthy body was one in perfect balance. Alcmaeon of Croton (about 500 BC), a pupil of Pythagoras, argued that a healthy body had the right balance of hot and cold, wet and dry within it. Any obvious imbalance (a high temperature or shivering) was a sign of ill health. The right treatment would be one which put the body back in balance.

We know very little about Hippocrates himself. He is associated with a collection of medical books, the *Hippocratic Corpus*. We do not know if he wrote any of the books himself, but they were written by his followers. Their importance is in showing us, for the first time, Greek medical thought. It is clear that there was a shift in emphasis at the time from concentrating on the illness to concentrating on the patient. Hippocrates did not want doctors to rely on a theory of the cause of disease that could be applied to every case, nor to depend on religious practices. Instead he wanted doctors to observe each patient and the progress of their illness carefully. He firmly rejected magical causes and cures. This system of observing the patient, which was something the Egyptians had also adopted, was developed into what we now call clinical observation.

Hippocrates emphasized the careful noting of symptoms. This was to help predict what would happen if another patient had the same disease. If there was a pattern in the development of a disease, the doctor would know what would happen next. Hippocrates believed it was important to let illness follow its natural course and provide

CLINICAL OBSERVATION

Clinical observation is the careful noting of all the symptoms of a disease and of the changes in the patient's condition during the course of an illness. A doctor was supposed to follow four steps.

Diagnosis
The doctor should study the symptoms of the patient. In what ways is the patient different from normal?

Prognosis
The doctor should try to predict what course the illness will follow. This should be done by thinking about previous patients with the same symptoms.

Observation
The doctor should then continue to observe the patients, noting changes in their condition and comparing them to the prognosis.

Treatment
The doctor should treat the patient, but only when his observations have confirmed his prognosis and he feels confident about the treatment to use from previous experience.

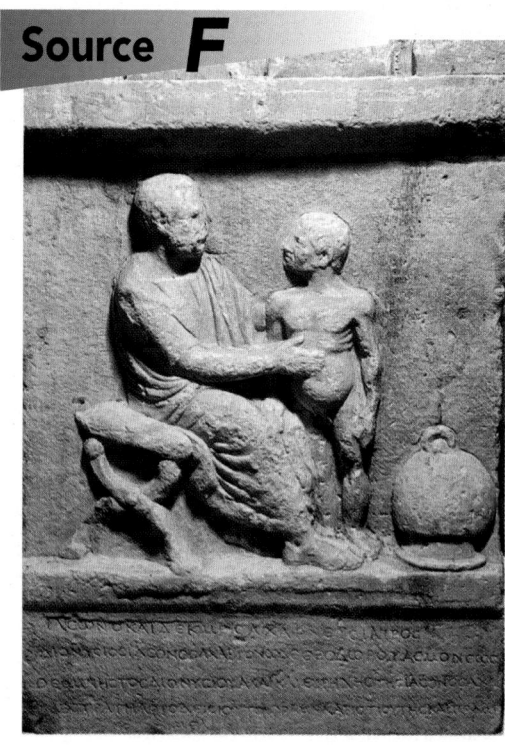

▶ The tombstone of Jason, an Athenian doctor, who died in the 2nd century AD. Jason is shown examining a patient. To the right (shown much larger than lifesize) is a bronze bleeding cup. It was heated, then placed over a small cut, and then cooled. This created a small vacuum which drew out some blood.

Source F

the patient with a clean and calm environment. A doctor could apply natural herbal remedies, but only once he was sure what was going on. But there were times when it was not possible simply to allow an illness to follow its natural course, when doctors had to resort to surgery.

Surgery in Greek times was dangerous. Because dissection was not allowed, doctors had only a vague idea about anatomy. They knew roughly where the internal organs were but had no idea of the way in which the circulation of the blood or the nervous system worked. The surgical Hippocratic books dealt mainly with the sort of procedures that had the highest success rate – the setting of fractures and the resetting of dislocated bones.

Source G

Quinsey has the symptoms of shivering, headache, swelling under the jaw, dry mouth. The patient found it hard to spit, or breathe lying down. He was bled from the first vertebra of the spine. He had to breathe a mixture of vinegar, soda, organy and watercress pounded together then mixed with oil and water and heated. He breathed it through a hollow reed, while hot sponges were applied to his jaw and neck. He gargled with herbs and had his throat cleaned out with a ball of wool on the end of a twig of myrtle.

▲ A description of symptoms and treatment given in a book in the Hippocratic collection called *On Diseases*.

4.4 The four humours

The Hippocratic books concentrate on observation. There is less material on treatment than on the symptoms of disease and the course a disease was likely to take. There is little about the cause of disease. The Hippocratic books sometimes talk about the body being made up of different elements, and the need for the elements to be in balance in a healthy person. The Greek tradition, however, was to try to work out complete theories about things. A later Greek thinker, Aristotle (384–322 BC), collected these ideas together and produced a clear statement of a theory about the cause and treatment of disease.

He suggested that the body was made up of four liquids or humours – blood, phlegm, yellow bile and black bile. There were also four seasons and these humours were connected to the seasons. Yellow bile was connected with the summer, black bile with the autumn, and so on. This meant it was possible there would be too much of the connected humour in the body in a particular season – too much phlegm in winter for instance. This was a problem because Aristotle believed that, to be healthy, a person needed to keep the humours in perfect balance. Here the careful observations of the Greek

doctors must have helped shape the theory. Some illnesses, like colds and bronchial problems are more common in winter than summer. These illnesses are likely to produce lots of phlegm. In the theory of the four humours this imbalance was seen as a *cause* of disease not a *symptom*. Doctors had to treat the patient and restore the balance between the humours. So, a patient who was feverish and hot probably had too much blood in his body. The solution was to 'bleed' the patient – take out blood by cutting into a vein.

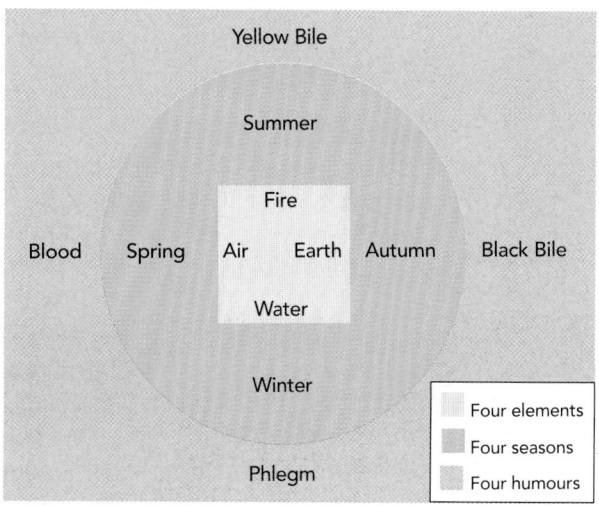

▲ The four humours.

Between 334 and 326 BC, Alexander the Great conquered a vast empire which stretched from Greece to Egypt and as far as India. In 332 BC he founded a new capital city, Alexandria, in Egypt. Soon after the great library of Alexandria was built with the intention of collecting all the knowledge of the world. It was stacked with the works of famous doctors, writers and philosophers.

Knowledge of anatomy could only **progress** when human dissection became acceptable. Philosophers like Plato and Aristotle argued that, once the soul of a person had left the body when he or she died, it was acceptable to cut the body up. This meant that people could gain a more accurate idea of the position of organs in the human body. They could examine the veins and arteries, muscles and bones.

Dissection was allowed in Alexandria – for a short time even dissection of the living was carried out. Criminals, who were condemned to die, were dissected and consequently the movement of blood around the veins was discovered. This practice was soon stopped. But dissection of the dead was still carried out, and advances in anatomy were made. The work carried out at Alexandria stressed accurate observation of what was actually there.

Herophilus (about 335–280 BC) worked in Alexandria on the comparative anatomy between men and animals. He also studied the nervous system, and worked out how it connected to the brain. However, he saw the nerves as channels to carry *pneuma* (the life force), not nervous impulses. Erasistratus (about 250 BC) wrote on anatomy and health. He was a very methodical anatomist, noticing the difference between arteries, veins and nerves. He thought, at first, that the nerves carried *pneuma* (like Herophilus), but then rejected this idea when he found that nerves were solid not hollow.

Because of the advances in anatomy, surgeons had a better idea of how the human body functioned, but this did not mean that surgery was much safer. There were still no anaesthetics or antibiotics, and hygiene was very poor. Unless they had a simple problem, patients were more likely to die than not.

Alexandria was famous for its study of surgery and medicine. Doctors who had studied there went to practise all over the world. But after the first few years, teachers and students split into various groups supporting the theories of the earlier writers. They developed competing theories of medicine and were more concerned with finding evidence to support their favourite theories than with studying what was actually there.

Source H

Chest trouble is heralded by sweating, a salty bitter matter in the mouth, unaccountable pains in the ribs and shoulder blades, trembling hands and dry coughs. They (the patients) should be treated with a mixture of radishes, cardamons, mustard, purslane and rocket pounded together and mixed with warm water. These will cause an easy and healing vomiting.

▲ From a book written by Diocles, a Greek doctor who lived in the 4th century BC.

QUESTIONS

1 Was Hippocratic medicine a change or a development? Explain your answer.

2 A doctor who accepted the theory of the four humours might bleed a patient. What would this doctor see as the cause of the problem and in which season of the year would the doctor be happiest doing this treatment?

3 In what way was medical practice in Alexandria a development on Hippocrates' work?

4 Explain how each of the following helped improve medicine at some time during the Greek period.

  a religion
  b a powerful central government.

Source I

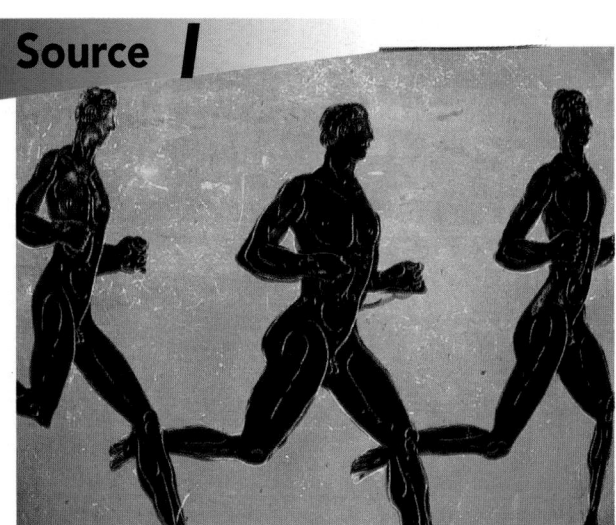

▲ A vase painting from 333 BC showing young men racing. Athletic exercise was thought to help people stay healthy.

Regimen was a word the Greeks used a lot when they discussed people's health. It covered all the aspects of their lives – what they ate or drank, how much they slept, how much exercise they took, what they did as a job. Everything was taken into account. The modern word would probably be 'lifestyle'.

Healthy habits

The idea of a regimen for a healthy life was not a new one. The Greeks had always believed that eating and drinking well helped to keep people healthy. Exercise and keeping clean had always been an important part of Greek life. The Hippocratic collection of books contained many titles that set out exactly what should be eaten, drunk, or avoided for perfect health, and when meals should be taken. They also outlined the best forms and amount of exercise to take. The advice about hygiene, eating and exercise, if fully followed, would have filled a normal day. Doctors seem to have realized that these were ideal measures which only the rich could take, and gave more general advice for ordinary people who had to work and therefore had restrictions on the time and money they could spend on their regimen.

Source J

After waking, a man should not get up at once but should wait until the heaviness of sleep has gone. After rising, he should rub his body with oil. He should then wash his hands, face and eyes with pure water. Thereafter he should, every day, wash his face and eyes with the hands using pure water. He should rub his teeth inside and out with his fingers, using fine peppermint powder to clean the teeth and remove the remains of food. He should oil his nose and ears, preferably with perfumed oil and rub oil into his hair every day, washing and combing it only at intervals.

After such a morning toilet, people who have to work, or choose to work will do so, but people of leisure will first take a walk. Long walks before meals clear out the body, prepare it for receiving food, and give it more power for digesting.

▲ From a book by Diocles, a Greek doctor of the 4th century BC.

Source K

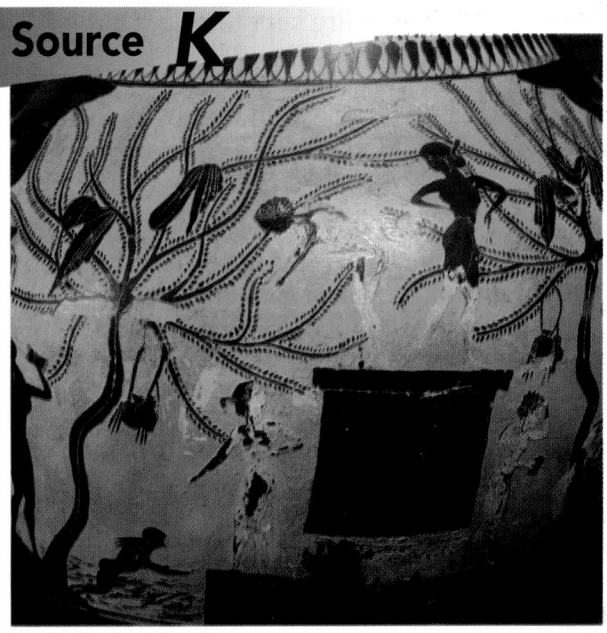

▶ A vase painting, from about 450 BC showing women washing.

CHAPTER 5

ROMAN MEDICINE

5.1 Roman civilization

Rome first conquered the rest of Italy, then most of the Mediterranean world. By 275 BC Rome had conquered the Greek cities in Italy; soon after the cities of mainland Greece fell. Rome was, from the first, a state which wanted to expand. It ruled a growing empire from Rome. Roman rule was efficient and centralized. Decisions were made in Rome, or referred to Rome for approval. Once made,

they were carried out by governors of the provinces and civil servants backed by a powerful army. It was vital to keep this army healthy. Like the Greeks and the Egyptians, the Romans were great builders but their work was more practical. Roman building achievements included aqueducts, sewers, roads and bridges rather than temples and monuments to the dead.

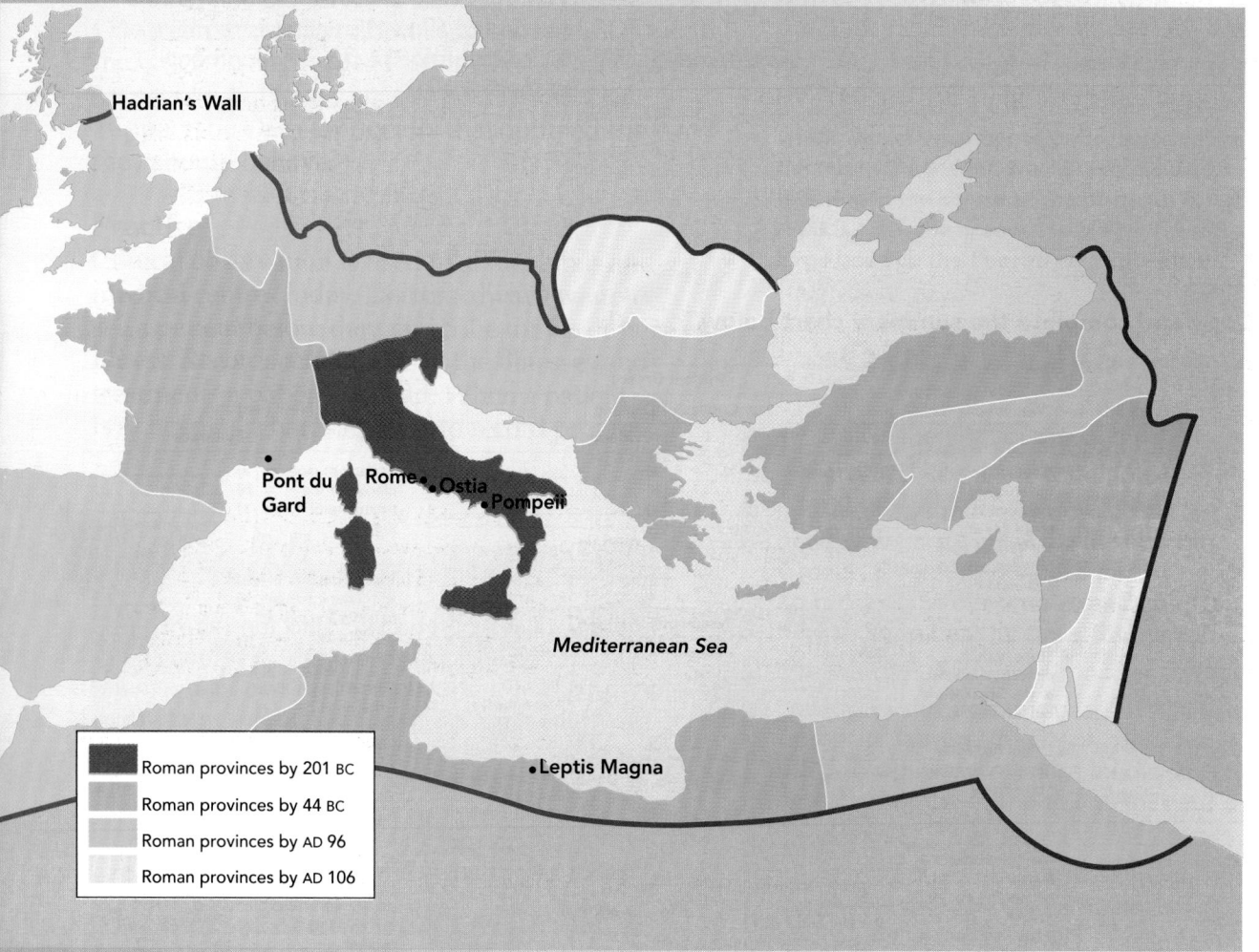

Hadrian's Wall

Pont du Gard

Rome
Ostia
Pompeii

Mediterranean Sea

Leptis Magna

Roman provinces by 201 BC
Roman provinces by 44 BC
Roman provinces by AD 96
Roman provinces by AD 106

▲ The Roman Empire.

5.2 Medicine in early Rome

In the early years, there were very few doctors in Rome. The head of each household was supposed to treat all the other people in it. The treatments were probably a mixture of common-sense and traditional superstition. Specialized medical knowledge was associated with the Greeks. Since the Romans had conquered Greece, Greeks had a very low social status, so doctors, who tended to be Greeks and were often slaves or ex-slaves, were not well thought of.

During an outbreak of plague in 293 BC the Romans founded an Asclepion in Rome itself, importing a sacred snake from the Asclepion at Epidaurus. Sited on an island in the Tiber, this continued to be a centre for the treatment of the sick throughout the Roman period. It was a public hospital where poor people and slaves could be treated.

The Romans wanted their whole population to be healthy. Apart from anything else, they needed to be able to recruit healthy soldiers. They appointed public doctors in Rome, and throughout the empire. These men were paid by the state, and treated the poor. As the army spread out to garrison the growing empire, hospitals for wounded soldiers (called *valetudinaria*) were

Source A

They have sworn to kill all barbarians with their drugs, and they call us barbarians. Remember that I forbid you to use doctors.

▲ The Roman writer Cato, who died in 149 BC, warning his son against Greek doctors. Cato treated his own family with cabbage, either externally, eaten, or mixed with wine.

QUESTIONS

1 List three characteristics of Roman civilization.

2 Are these similar to, or different from, the main characteristics of Greek civilization?

3 The Egyptians and the Greeks both made some doctors into gods and respected all doctors; in Rome this was not usually the case. Does this mean the Romans did not think medicine was very important?

4 Rome had a well-organized government which was efficient at raising taxes. Did this have any effect on Roman medicine?

Source B

Social and ethnic status of Roman doctors from the 1st to the 3rd century AD

	Total	Greek	Greek %
Citizens	186	118	63
Freedmen	170	158	93
Slaves	55	54	98
Foreign, non-citizens	31	23	74
Total	442	353	80

◀ This table lists all the doctors for whom tombstones have been found. Obviously this is only a small fraction of the number of doctors there would have been in those 300 years. Based on figures in V. Nutton, *A Social History of Graeco-Roman Medicine*.

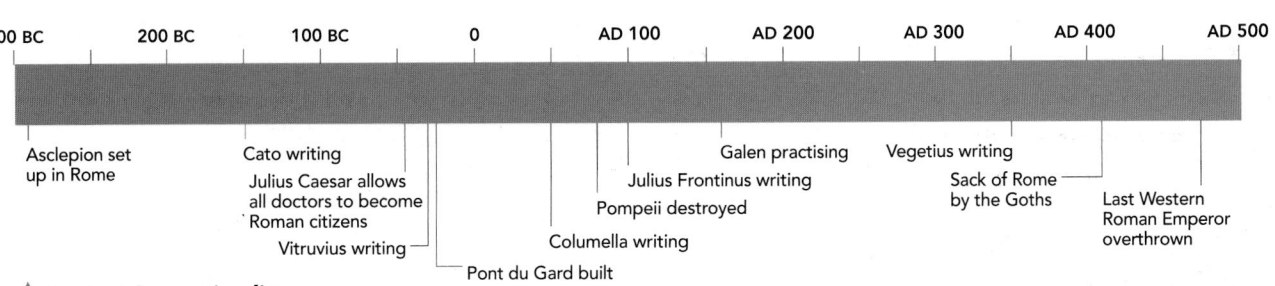

300 BC — 200 BC — 100 BC — 0 — AD 100 — AD 200 — AD 300 — AD 400 — AD 500

Asclepion set up in Rome

Cato writing

Julius Caesar allows all doctors to become Roman citizens

Vitruvius writing

Pont du Gard built

Columella writing

Pompeii destroyed

Julius Frontinus writing

Galen practising

Vegetius writing

Sack of Rome by the Goths

Last Western Roman Emperor overthrown

▲ Ancient Rome timeline.

set up. Because they were popular, others were set up for the civil servants who governed the empire and, then, still more to treat poor people and slaves who worked on farms.

Doctors were still seen as having low social status. However, in 46 BC Julius Caesar passed a decree allowing them to become Roman citizens, and those who successfully treated the wealthy and powerful could become famous and wealthy themselves. Greeks came to dominate the profession throughout the Roman period.

5.3 Public health

For the Romans prevention was better than cure. However, before they could prevent illness they had to decide what caused it. The Romans were a very practical people and they learnt much from observation. One of the things they observed was that people who lived near marshes and swamps tended to get ill, and often die from the disease we now call malaria. Was there a connection between the swamps and the illness? The first solution was to build a temple to Febris the goddess of fever in the largest swamp near Rome. If you believe in supernatural causes and cures for disease, this is the obvious thing to do. However, over time, they must have noticed that there were just as many people dying as before. The next attempt to solve the problem was to drain the swamps. The fewer swamps there were near Rome the less malaria there would be. It worked.

Empirical observation

This shows two very important things about the Roman system of public health.

- It could only work within the Romans' understanding of the causes of disease. However, sharp observation and common-sense could get them a long way. They realized the swamp was part of the problem, while not knowing the way in which mosquitoes spread malaria. This **empirical** method of solving problems, acting on what they knew was happening rather than waiting until they knew exactly why it was happening, was often used by the Romans.

- The Romans were willing to tackle large engineering projects in order to solve problems. Draining the swamps around Rome cannot have been cheap or easy, but the Romans had the will-power, the resources, and the technology to do it.

Their empirical observations suggested to the Romans that a number of things were likely to cause disease:

- bad smells or 'bad air'
- bad water
- swamps and marshes
- being near sewage
- not keeping clean.

They made sure they took all these things into account when choosing a site for a house, a new town, or a military camp. They also worked hard to get rid of these problems in the great towns and cities they had already built.

Source C

The new Anio aqueduct is taken from the river which is muddy and discoloured because of the ploughed fields on either side. Because of this a special filter tank was placed at the start of the aqueduct where soil could settle and the water clarify before going along the channel.

▲ Julius Frontinus, the Curator of Rome's water supply, writing about AD 100.

Source D

There should be no marshes near buildings, for marshes give off poisonous vapours during the hot period of the summer. At this time they give birth to animals with mischief-making stings which fly at us in thick swarms.

▲ Columella, a Roman writer, who lived in the 1st century AD. At one time he had been a soldier but spent most of his life as a farmer and a writer of books on country life.

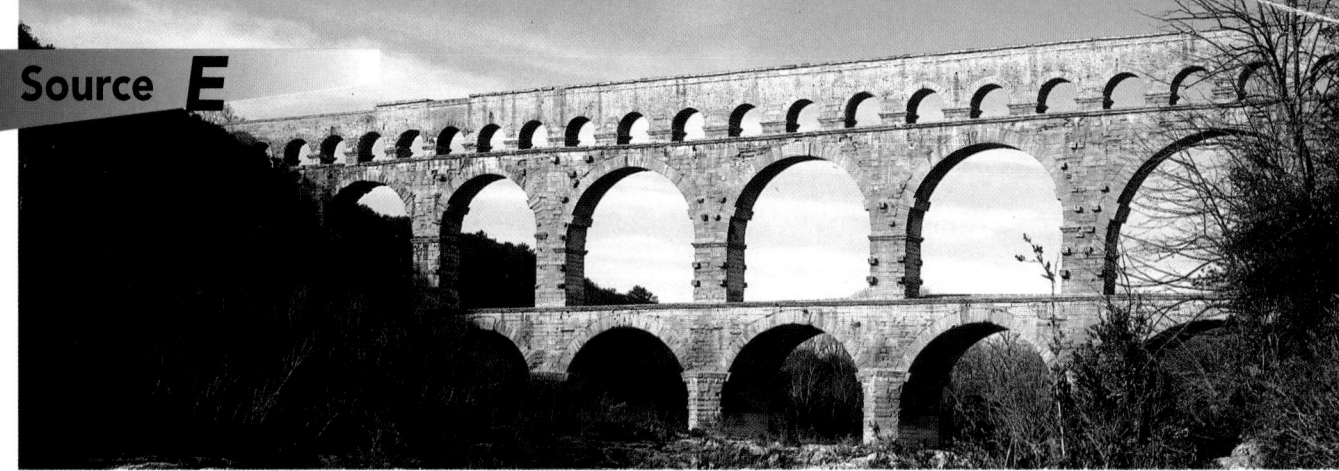

Source E

▲ The Pont du Gard aqueduct, which carried water from Uzes to the Roman town at Nîmes in southern France.

Source F

We must take great care in searching for springs and, in selecting them, keeping in mind the health of the people. If a spring runs free and open, look carefully at the people who live nearby before beginning to pipe the water. If their bodies are strong, their complexions fresh, their legs sound and eyes clear then the water is good. If this water is boiled in a bronze cauldron without any sand or mud left in the bottom of the cauldron, then the water will be excellent.

▲ Vitruvius, a Roman writer and architect who lived in the 1st century BC.

Source G

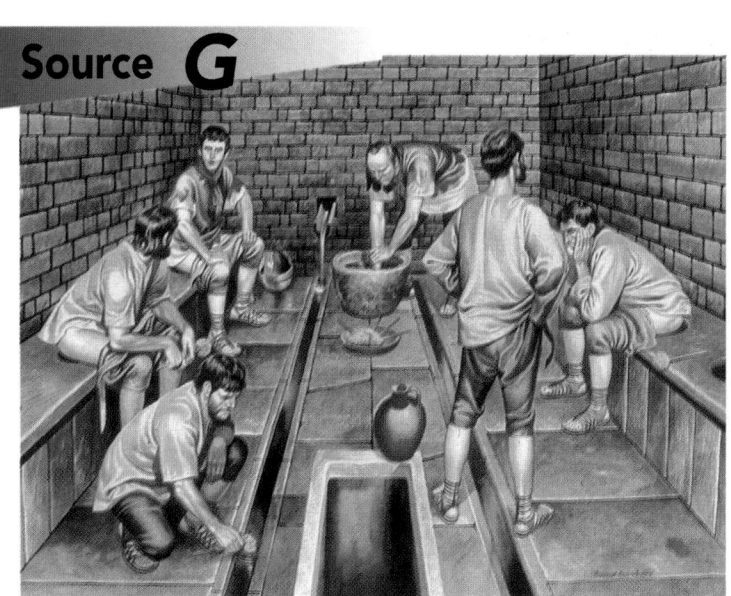

▲ A modern artist's reconstruction of a toilet on Hadrian's Wall. Water ran through a channel under the seats to clean the sewage. Clean water ran through the channels in front of the seats.

Source H

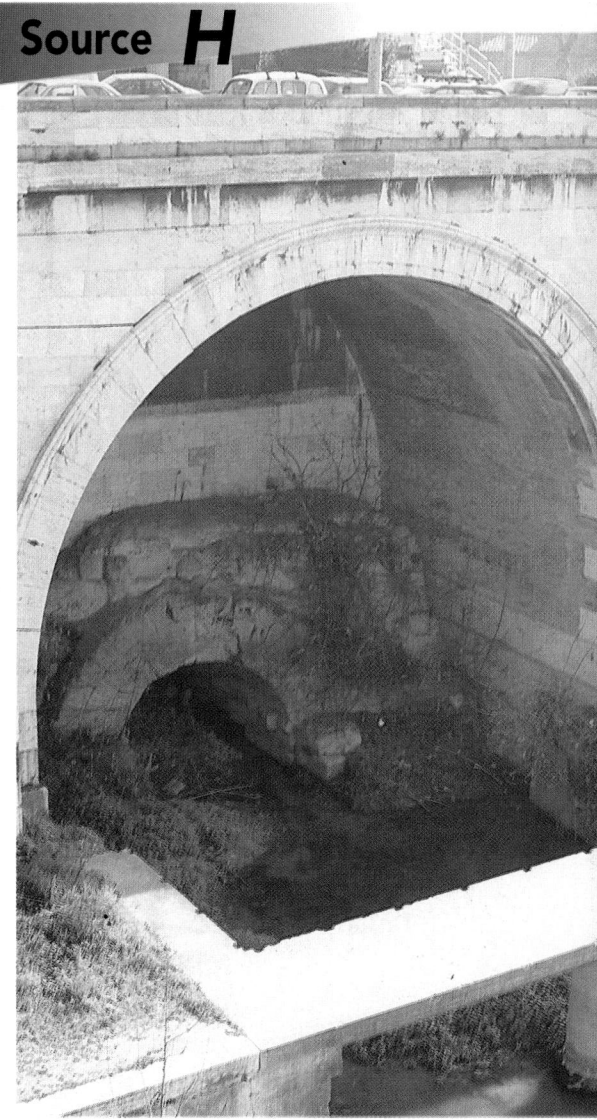

▲ The smaller inner arch is the original outlet of Rome's main sewer, the *Cloaca Maxima*, into the River Tiber. From the water to the top of the arch is over 2 metres.

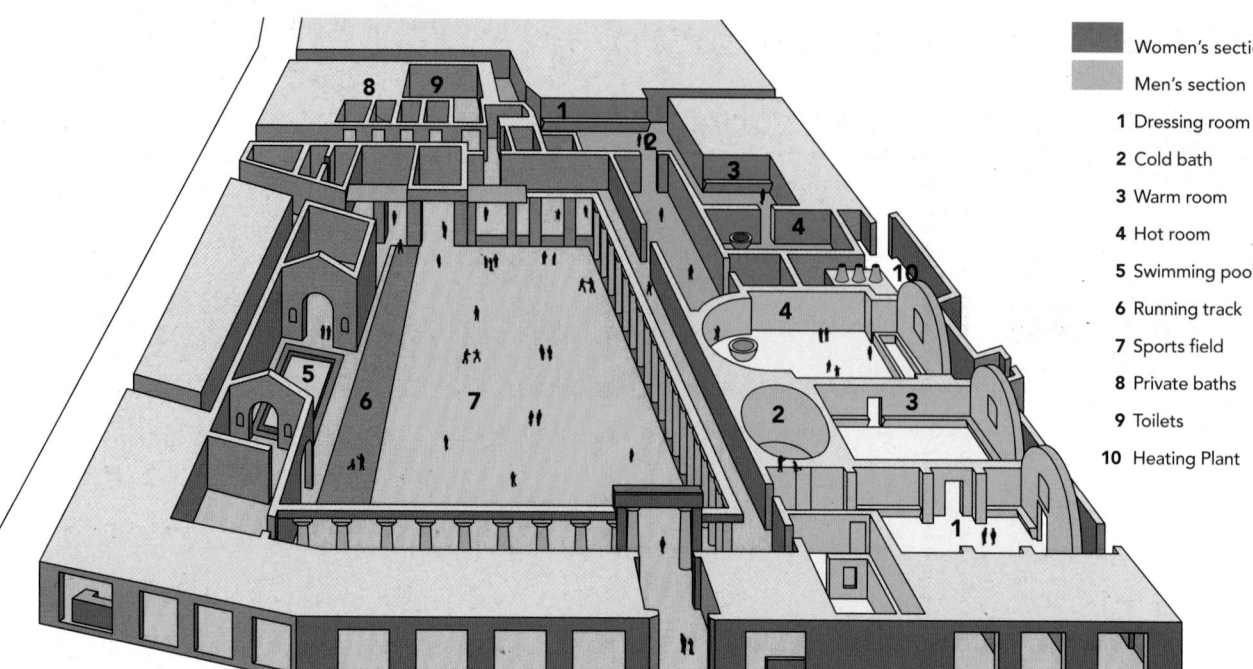

▲ Stabian Baths at Pompeii.

Women's section

Men's section

1 Dressing room
2 Cold bath
3 Warm room
4 Hot room
5 Swimming pool
6 Running track
7 Sports field
8 Private baths
9 Toilets
10 Heating Plant

Aqueducts

The Romans used their engineering skills to bring pure water into their towns. There were 14 aqueducts bringing 1350 million litres of fresh water a day into Rome. The water ran through brick and stone channels. The Romans had no system for pumping water, so the whole course of the channel had to run gently downwards. This meant that the channels usually started in the nearest hills or mountains. Valleys could be crossed by building aqueducts, while sometimes tunnels had to be cut through hills. When the water reached the cities it was used for many purposes.

Source

◄ The warm room of the men's section of the Stabian Baths.

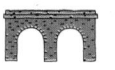

Emperor 17.1%

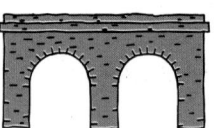

Private houses and industry 38.6%

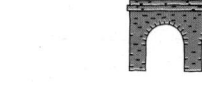

Military barracks 2.9%

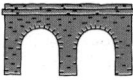

Official buildings 24.1%

Public buildings, baths and theatres 3.9%

Public cisterns and fountains 13.4%

▲ The way Rome's water supply was used in AD 100.

THE FORUM PUBLIC TOILETS, POMPEII

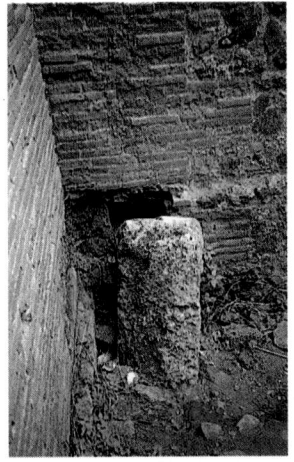

▲ The area marked a on the plan.

◀ A plan of the Forum public toilet (not to scale).

b

a   Inner door   c

Vestibule

Entrance

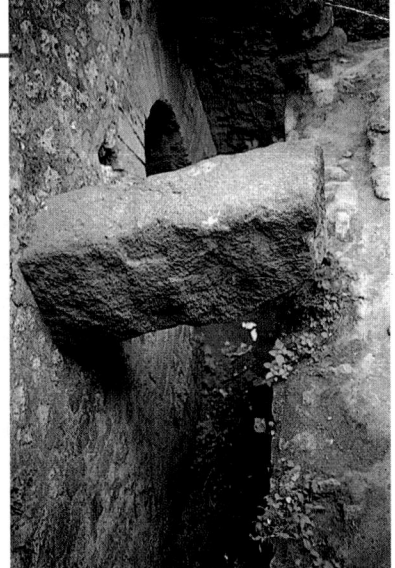

▲ The area marked b on the plan.

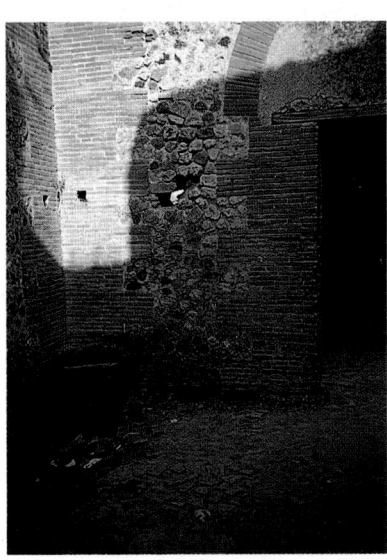

▲ The area marked c on the plan.

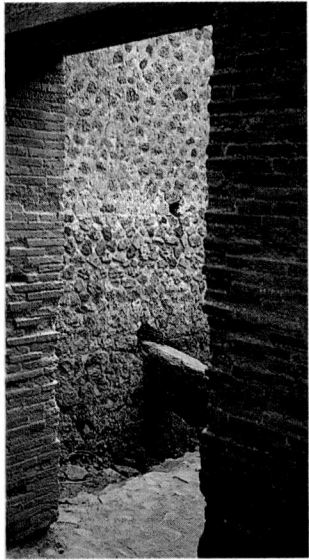

▲ Looking inside from the vestibule.

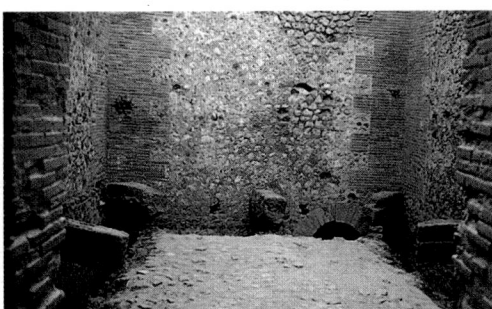

▲ The view from the inner door.

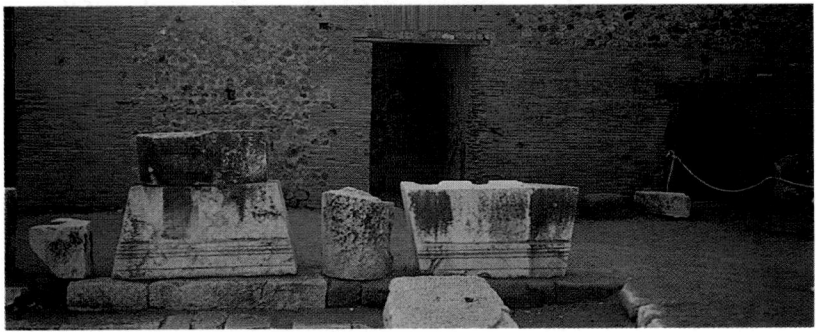

▲ The entrance to the men's toilet from the Forum.

Compare the Forum toilets in Pompeii with the reconstruction of the toilet on Hadrian's Wall (Source G, page 33).

What is shown at points **a**, **b** and **c** on the plan?

How was sewage taken out of the toilet?

What are the similarities and differences between this public toilet and modern ones?

Galen's study of the brain was undermined by his use of animals. He described a network of small blood vessels on the under-surface of the brain called the *rete mirabile* (the wonderful network). He gave this *rete mirabile* a very important place in his theory of how the body works. Unfortunately it is found only in certain animals and not in humans.

Galen's observation also let him down. He was convinced that there were minute holes in the *septum* which divides the two chambers of the heart. These holes play an important part in Galen's physiology, but there are, in fact, no such holes.

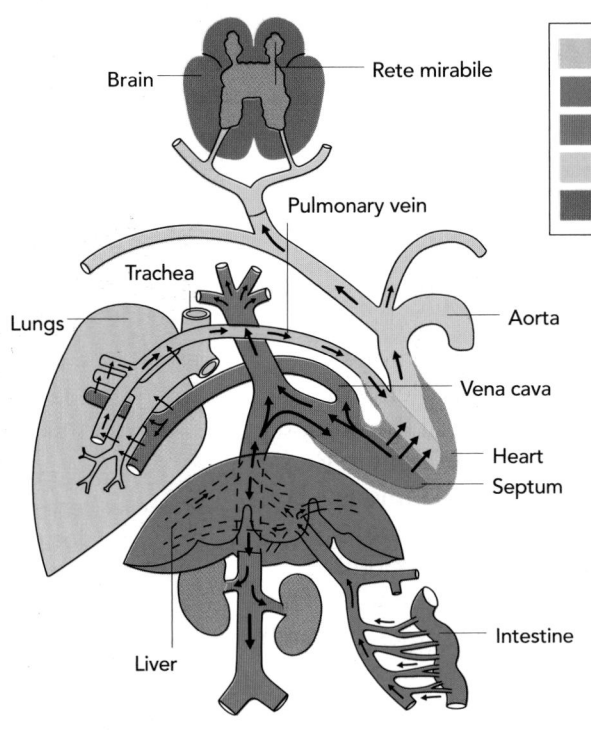

▲ **Galen's physiological system.**

	pneuma
	chyle
	blood with natural spirit
	blood with vital spirit
	blood with animal spirit

Pneuma (life-giving spirit) was breathed in, went from the lungs to the heart and mixed with the blood.

Chyle (the goodness from food) went from the intestines to the liver where it was made into blood with Natural Spirit.

Blood with Natural Spirit went throughout the body nourishing and enabling growth. From the heart some went to the lungs, and some passed through the septum where it mixed with the pneuma to form blood with Vital Spirit.

Blood with Vital Spirit went into the arteries giving power to the body. When this blood reached the brain it was changed into blood with Animal Spirit.

Blood with Animal Spirit went through the nerves (which Galen believed were hollow) to give the body sensation and motion.

Galen's importance

Galen was the ancient author who had the biggest influence on Arab and Christian doctors of the Middle Ages. There are a number of reasons for this. He drew on the work and ideas of all the great doctors since Hippocrates. He wrote many books, most of which survived. He wrote powerfully, always dealing with possible objections to his theories. In many ways, his writing was like a speech in a debate. Also, he provided a complete theory of medicine; his books dealt with diagnosis and treatment, surgery, anatomy and physiology. Perhaps even more important, although he was writing in the 2nd century AD when the Romans worshipped many gods, his theories were acceptable to Christians and Muslims who worshipped only one god. Galen often talked about *'the creator'* in his writing. He thought of the body as the work of a great architect or designer. This fitted in well with the religious beliefs which were to dominate Europe over the next 1,300 years.

QUESTIONS

1 Galen trained as a doctor in Pergamum and Alexandria. What is the significance of these two cities in the development of medicine in the Ancient World?

2 Galen's first job was as a doctor to gladiators. Why might this have given him some special advantages?

3 Explain, according to Galen's physiology, what happened to:

a pneuma

b food

c blood with natural spirit

d blood with vital spirit

e blood with animal spirit.

4 Should historians of medicine see Galen's work as a development or a change?

5 What effect did religious beliefs have on Galen's work?

6 Galen's theory of anatomy and physiology was wrong. Does this mean it is not important in the history of medicine?

5.6 Exercise

Study the following sources.

Source 1

When Marcus Agrippa was a government official in charge of the sewers he travelled under Rome in a boat. There are seven tunnels in the city which run into one great sewer. Swollen with the rain water they sweep away all the city's sewage.

*   *   *   *   *   *

Our forefathers condemned the medical profession. They refused to pay fees to profiteers in order to save their lives.

▲ From Pliny's *Natural History*, written in Rome about AD 50.

Source 2

The school of medicine founded by Hippocrates spread all over Greece from the 5th century BC onwards. His methods of observing and recording a patient's symptoms were scientific. The aim was to forecast accurately the course of an illness.

▲ Hugh Lloyd Jones, *The Greek World*, 1965.

1 How do the attitudes of the Greeks described in Source 1 differ from those of the Romans?

2 The Romans copied many Greek ideas but they had different attitudes to medicine. Why?

3 How important were each of the following in Greek and Roman medicine:

   a the power of governments

   b the ideas of great doctors

   c transport and communications?

Copy and complete the summary chart below.

Roman Medicine						
Factors affecting Medicine		**Causes of Disease**			**New Features**	
Factor	Effect	Cause	Evidence		Feature	Evidence
1 _____	Romans could not learn from the drainage and water supply ideas of the Minoans.	1 Spiritual	a) _____ b) Building a temple to Febris to stop fever in Rome.		1 Well developed public health system concentrating on preventing disease.	a) Aqueducts (eg Pont du Gard) b) _____ c) _____ d) Sewers (eg Cloaca Maxima in Rome)
2 _____	Large projects requiring complex organization and a lot of money could be undertaken like public baths and aqueducts.	2 Bad air, especially bad smells, associated with sewage and swamps.	a) _____ b) _____ c) _____			
		3 Bad water	a) _____ b) _____			
3 _____	Rome's interest in public health was partly because it wanted a healthy army.	4 Not keeping your body clean and fit.	_____		2 New ideas about human anatomy based on studying animals.	_____
4 _____	Beliefs did not allow human dissection which held back understanding of anatomy.					

Treatments Used		
Treatment	Illness	Evidence
1 Pepper	_____	Galen
2 Vigorous exercise	General weakness recovering from a major illness.	_____

CHAPTER 6

THE FALL OF THE ROMAN EMPIRE IN THE WEST

In the late 4th century AD the Roman Empire was in decline. Tribes of Huns, Goths and Vandals were threatening the Empire. There no longer seemed to be the power and drive within the Roman state to reform itself. In AD 395 the Empire split into two – an Eastern Empire ruled from Byzantium and a Western Empire ruled from Rome. The Western Empire was soon in trouble. In AD 410, the Goths invaded Italy and sacked Rome itself. In AD 476 the last Roman Emperor in the west was deposed by a Germanic chieftain.

By concentrating on Britain, we can see what the fall of the Roman Empire meant to ordinary people, and to medicine. The last Roman troops probably left Britain around AD 410 and the abandoned province was left to the mercy of the invading Saxons. With the breaking of the link with Rome, those features of life in Roman Britain which depended on a strong central government quickly fell into disrepair. Within a hundred years many Roman towns were either abandoned or became Saxon settlements. The water supply stopped working. The sewage system no longer worked. Houses no longer had sophisticated heating systems – a fire in the middle of the floor was more common. There were no more public or private baths. Most significant of all, the strong and stable Roman rule – known as the *Pax Romana* (Roman Peace) – had degenerated into something close to anarchy. In England there were a number of small British kingdoms, all fighting for survival against bands of Saxon invaders.

As a result of this upheaval knowledge was lost. Roman and Greek manuscripts were neglected and destroyed. People with the engineering skill to build, or even repair, the Roman public works died, and no new people were trained up in their place. Within a hundred years, people were living in a country where technology was much less advanced than it had been in their grandparents' time.

Source A

Well-wrought this wall: Wierds [fates] broke it
The stronghold burst...
Snapped rooftrees, towers fallen, the work of Giants, the stonesmiths, mouldereth.
And the wielders and wrights [workmen]? Earthgrip holds them – gone, long gone, fast in gravesgrasp.

▲ Part of an Anglo-Saxon poem, *The Ruin*, written in AD 700. It describes a ruined Roman city – probably Bath.

Source B

When you see a dung beetle throwing up earth, catch it and a handful of the earth between your hands. Wave it about vigorously and say:

'Remedium facio ad ventris dolorum' [Give relief to a painful stomach].

Then throw the beetle away over your back, take care not to look at it after this. When someone comes to you with a sore stomach, hold the stomach between your hands and they will soon be well. This will work for twelve months after catching the beetle.

▲ A Saxon remedy for stomach ache.

Source 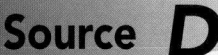 C

Catch a frog when neither moon or sun is shining, cut off the hind legs and wrap them in deerskin. Apply the frog's right leg to the right foot and the left leg to the left foot of the gouty patient and he will certainly be cured.

▲ A cure used by 'Gilbert' a doctor working in the early 11th century.

Source D

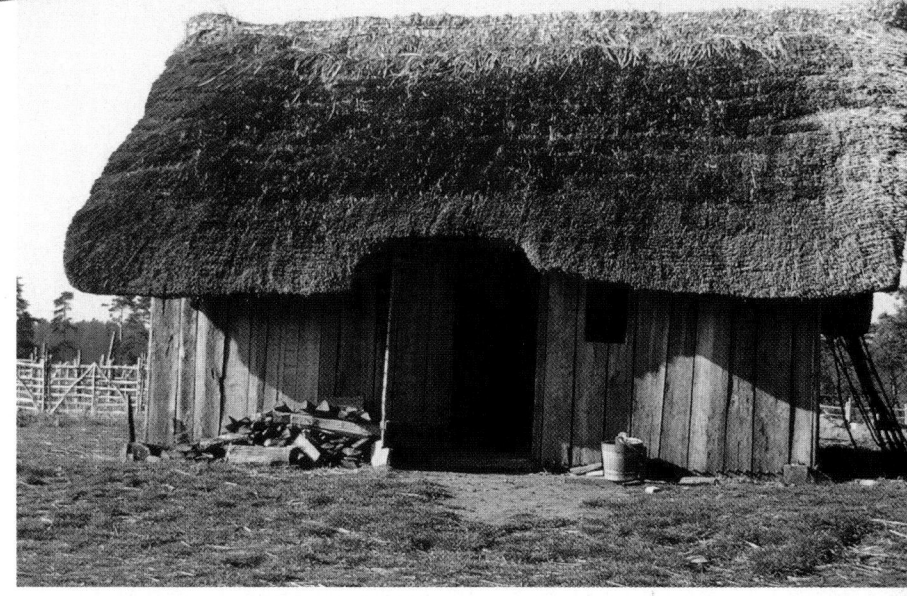

▲ A reconstruction of a Saxon home.

▼ The Dark Ages timeline.

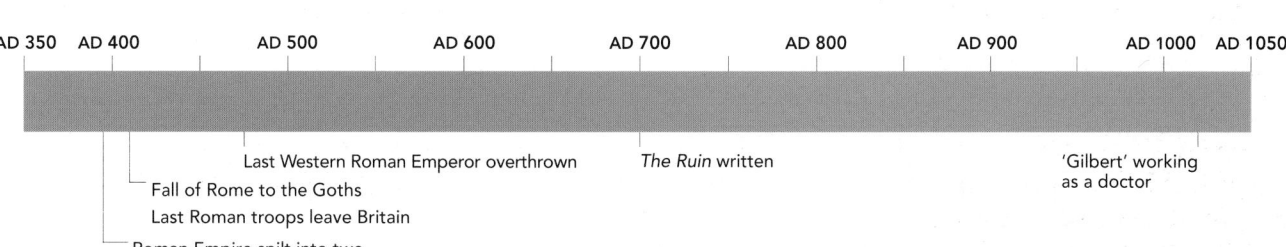

AD 350 AD 400 AD 500 AD 600 AD 700 AD 800 AD 900 AD 1000 AD 1050

Last Western Roman Emperor overthrown   *The Ruin* written   'Gilbert' working as a doctor

Fall of Rome to the Goths
Last Roman troops leave Britain
Roman Empire spilt into two

QUESTIONS

1 Who were the 'Giants' in Source A?

2 a How would you describe the belief about the causes of disease shown in Source B?

  b How would you describe the belief about the causes of disease shown in Source C?

3 Historians have sometimes called the period between AD 476 and about AD 850, The Dark Ages. Why do you think this is?

4 Did medicine in Britain progress or regress between about AD 400 and AD 800? Support your answer with both reference to sources and other facts about the history of medicine.

PROGRESS AND REGRESS

In this book we are looking at one aspect of human society, medicine, through time. We need to be careful how we use the technical words which describe the story. **Progress** means something moving forward. In our context getting better, improving. **Regress** means something moving backwards. In our case, getting worse.

CHAPTER 7

ORIENTAL MEDICINE — ISLAM AND CHINA

7.1 Islamic civilization

The Roman Empire in the West had collapsed by AD 500. Within a hundred years, a new civilization was growing up in the Middle East. This civilization was based around the teachings of Muhammad who was born in Arabia in AD 570. The new religion of Islam founded by Muhammad swept rapidly east, west and south until, by the year AD 1000, it covered parts of southern Asia, north Africa and southern Europe (see map). This whole area was united by the Islamic religion and the Arabic language. For a long time the capital of this empire was Baghdad.

The religion of Islam

The Holy Book of Islam is the *Qur'an*, an Arabic word which means 'recitation'. The *Qur'an* governs a Muslim's whole life for it describes how he or she should live. It includes the duties of parents to their children, of masters to their servants and of the rich to the poor. The roles of men and women are described, as are the duties regarding praying, fasting and pilgrimage.

The rule of the Abbasids

By AD 750 the Abbasids, a dynasty of Sultans who were descended from Muhammad's uncle, were ruling from Baghdad. They built a beautiful city that grew to a size of 8 kilometres across. It contained hundreds of mosques, fine buildings and public baths. The wealth of the city came from trade with places as far afield as China, India, Russia, Spain and Africa. Leather, silk, furs, silver and spices flowed into Baghdad and with them came knowledge and new ideas and learning from distant lands. For the next 500 years, the Abbasids ruled from Baghdad. Although they did not remain powerful all the time, Arabic remained the common language throughout the empire and Islam the main religion. Wherever they settled in new lands, the Muslims set up schools and built mosques. Later, universities were founded.

QUESTIONS

1 What is the *Qur'an* and what does it mean to a Muslim?

2 What common features helped to unite the Arab Empire?

3 What were the similarities between Baghdad in AD 750 and Rome when the Roman Empire was at its most powerful?

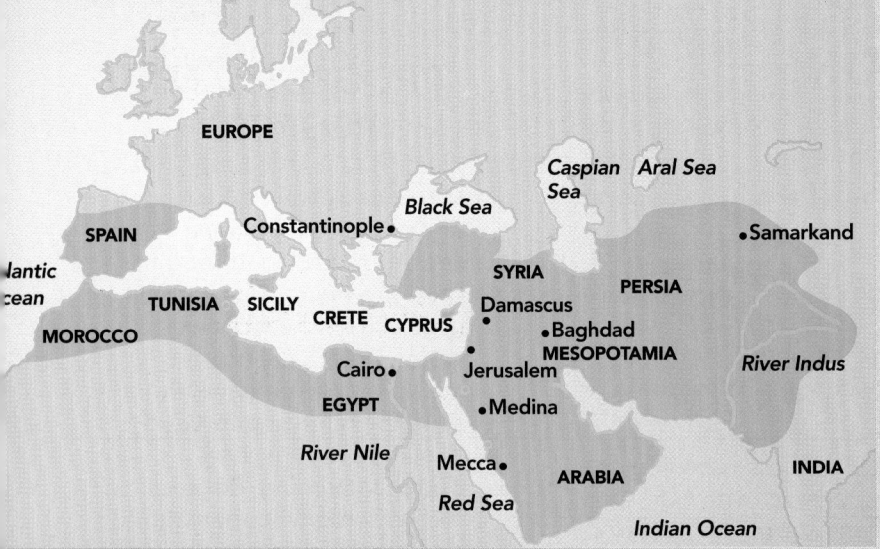

Islamic influence in about AD 1000.

Whilst the Roman Empire in the West was destroyed by invasions of barbarians, the Eastern Empire had survived. This meant that the learning of the ancient Greeks and Romans had been preserved. The Greek speaking scholars of the Eastern Empire still read, used and sometimes translated the works of the ancient authors on mathematics, astronomy and medicine.

Nestorius

From the Eastern Empire these medical ideas had spread to neighbouring countries. In AD 431, the Christian Patriarch of Jerusalem, Nestorius, had been banished for heresy. He and his followers moved eastwards, finally settling in Jundi Shapur in Persia, where they set up a famous medical centre. At the same time, Nestorius and his Christian followers translated the ancient Greek medical texts like the Hippocratic Corpus and Galen's works into Arabic.

The spread of Islamic influence

Just over a hundred years later, Muhammad was born and, as we have seen, in the next century, Islamic influence spread rapidly. Although the names 'Arab' and 'Arabian' are usually given to the scientists and translators in the Arab Empire because they worked and spoke in Arabic, very few at this time were actually Arabs. Like Nestorius and his followers, they might have been Christians, or perhaps Jews, and could have come from many different parts of the Islamic world like Syria or Persia. They were united by using the Arab language and by living within this growing Arab Empire around the Mediterranean Sea.

Source B

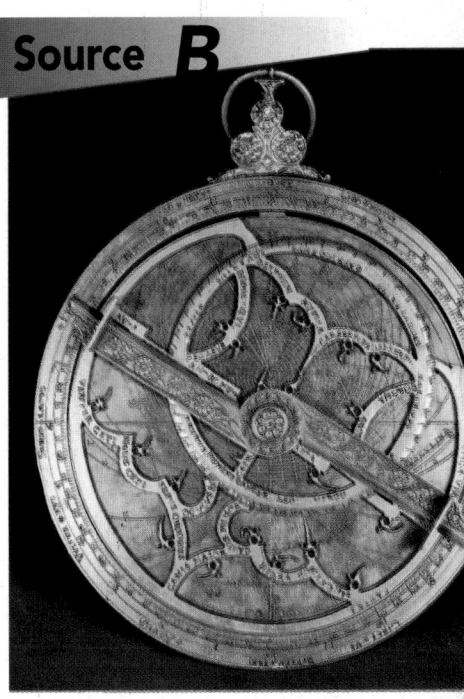

► The astrolabe is believed to have been invented by a Greek named Hipparchus in 150 BC. Islamic scholars developed the instrument and it became the chief aid to navigation for many centuries. This one dates from the 16th century AD.

By the 8th and 9th centuries AD the Arab world had become a centre for learning and new ideas. Hunain ibn Ishaq (known as Johannitius) spent two years travelling in Greece and collecting Greek texts. He returned to Baghdad and commented on and translated many of these books, including the works of Hippocrates and Galen, into Arabic. He died, chief of the physicians in Baghdad, in AD 873. By 1100 the same works were translated into Latin (probably in Toledo in Spain). In this way, Greek learning was preserved.

Source A

In the 9th and 10th centuries, Cordoba was a city of 200,000 houses, 600 mosques and 900 public baths. Its streets were paved and water was piped to the people. Its library had 600,000 books and there were 50 other libraries in the region.

▲ Hugh Thomas, *Spain*, 1964.

QUESTIONS

1 How did the work of the Greek and Roman authors pass into the Islamic world?

2 What part did chance play in the transmission of these ideas?

Causes of disease

In Muhammad's time many Arab doctors believed that illness was caused by the evil spirits. However, as a result of reading the books by doctors such as Galen and Hippocrates, they adopted many of the theories about diagnosing illness through an understanding of the four humours and the need to keep a balance of humours within the body (see page 25).

As important, however, was the fact that they adopted Hippocrates' methods of observation. He had said that it was vitally important to watch a sick patient closely to note every detail of skin colour, rash, cough, temperature and so on. Doctors such as Rhazes took this to heart. He was a Persian who became senior doctor at one of the Baghdad hospitals in about AD 900. He was the first to observe and write about the differences between smallpox and measles. His greatest work was his huge book *al-Hawi* (the comprehensive book).

Perhaps the greatest doctor and author of over a hundred books was Avicenna (AD 980–1037). He, too, was a Persian and a brilliant scholar. Before he was ten-years old he could recite the whole *Qur'an* from memory. When he was eighteen years old, he became the doctor to the **caliphs** in Baghdad. He is said to have shortened his life by indulging in too much wine and high living, but even so, he wrote the most famous and probably the most influential medical book ever. This book, the *Canon of Medicine*, lays out a complete system of medicine based on the work of Galen but also includes new facts and observations drawn from Avicenna's own experience.

This work was influential for two reasons. Firstly, it was excellent and is still worth reading by modern doctors. Secondly, it was translated into Latin and, therefore, brought the ideas of Galen back into Western Europe where it was the main textbook used by medical students until about 1700.

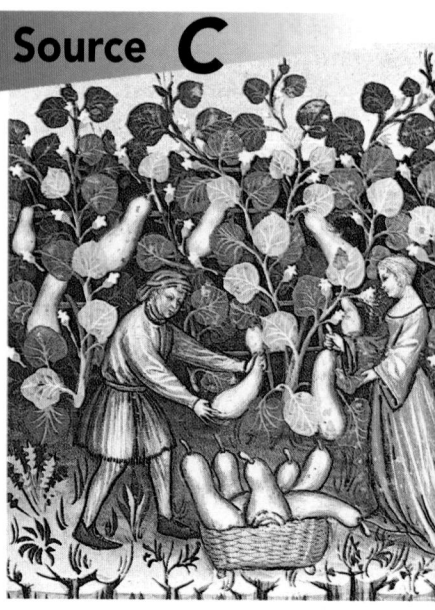

Source C

▲ An Arabic manuscript written by a doctor in Baghdad in the 11th century. It shows people harvesting marrows which were used to cleanse the bowels and to quench thirst.

Source D

The main symptoms of smallpox are backache, fever, stinging pains, redness of the cheeks and eyes and difficulty with breathing.

Excitement, nausea and unrest are more pronounced in measles than they are in smallpox, while aching in the back is less.

▲ From *On Smallpox and Measles*, written by Rhazes, a Persian doctor, in about AD 900.

QUESTIONS

1 What evidence is there that at least some Arab doctors developed Hippocrates' insistence on close observation of sick patients?

2 a Describe the work of Rhazes.
  b Describe the work of Avicenna.
  c Which was more important in the development of medicine? Give reasons for your answer.

Hospitals

Medicine was well organized. By AD 850 Baghdad had its first hospital and by AD 931, doctors in the city had to pass examinations to obtain a licence. Other hospitals were set up throughout the Muslim world, the most famous being in Damascus and Cairo.

Surgery

The greatest Arab surgeon was Albucasis who was born in Cordoba, in Spain, in about AD 936. He was obviously a careful and painstaking man. He advised surgeons only to operate when they knew the cause of the pain and always to work out first what they were going to do. He also warned that Allah was watching and the surgeon should never operate for personal gain. He wrote about amputations, lithotomy (removing stones from the bladder) and dentistry (putting in artificial teeth made of bone). He described how to sew wounds, how to set fractures and deal with dislocations.

Anatomy

Dissecting human bodies was forbidden by Islamic Law, so Arab doctors could not check on Galen's description of the bones and soft tissues of the body. The only real criticism of Galen came from Ibn an-Nafis, a doctor in Cairo during the 13th century. Making his own observations, he said (correctly) that blood did not pass through the septum (see p.38).

Chemistry

Perhaps the greatest overall Arab contribution to learning was in chemistry. They invented many processes such as **distillation** and **sublimation** – both used in the preparation of drugs. They also added some drugs to general use such as laudanum, senna, musk, benzoin and camphor.

Source E

In the Cairo hospital, founded in 1283, there were special divisions for the wounded, for eye patients, for those with fever (in whose rooms the air was refreshed with fountains) and for gynaecological cases. The convalescent received at his departure five pieces of gold that he might not be obliged to return to work immediately.

▲ W. J. Bishop, *The Early History of Surgery*, 1960.

Source F

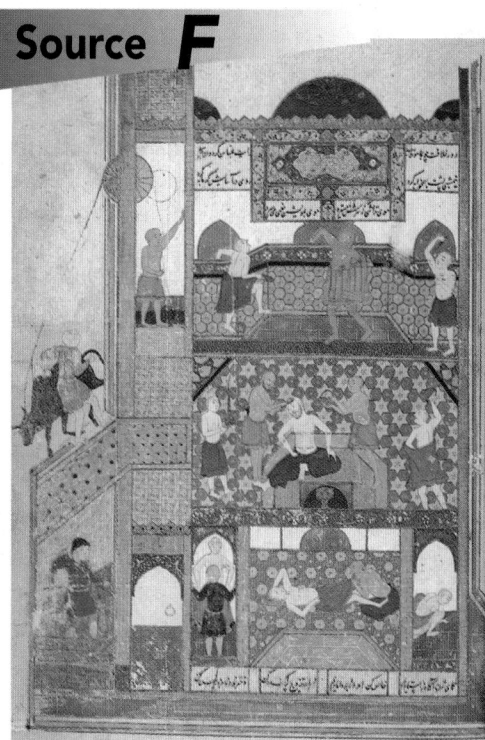

▲ Caliph Manum (AD 813–33) having a shower, haircut and massage in the bath-house of his palace in Baghdad.

QUESTIONS

1 a Describe the new features of Islamic medicine.
  b What continuity was there between Islamic medicine and Greek and Roman medicine?

2 Ibn an-Nafis' work on the septum was unknown in Europe until 1924. Is this significant in the development of medicine?

For thousands of years China was geographically isolated from the Western world. This meant that its civilization developed on unique lines.

By about 200 BC, Inner China was united under the rule of the first emperor of the Qin dynasty, a fearsome dictator. The unity of China did not last for long for his son was just as harsh but not as clever. From years of civil war, a new leader emerged – the first emperor of the Han dynasty. This dynasty lasted for about 400 years (206 BC–AD 220) before China fell apart into warring states again. This was to be a recurring pattern for China for hundreds of years.

Government in China

Throughout all this time there was a continuous thread of well organized government. The emperors set up government departments for taxation, trade, famine control, irrigation, medicine, astronomy and so on. Thus there were thousands of civil servants both in the capital and all over China, gathering taxes, running law courts, overseeing irrigation and running the government owned industries. By 120 BC, all iron production was carried on in 49 government run factories scattered throughout the empire.

The Silk Road

The only real contact with India and the West was along the Silk Road. It was along this route that China's technological achievements such as the making of paper, silk, gunpowder, wheelbarrows and windmills reached the West. In return China absorbed ideas such as Buddhist teachings from India which influenced Chinese thinking and medicine over the centuries. But the contact was always limited.

Source G

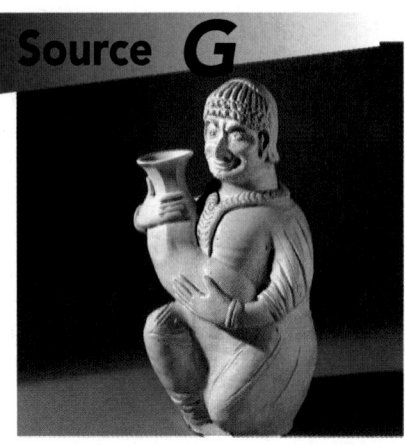

▲ A pottery figure of a foreign merchant. The Chinese called such people foreign devils and found the round eyes, big noses and lighter hair of outsiders both ugly and fascinating. They were convinced that everyone outside China was a barbarian.

QUESTIONS

1 Write a short account of the Chinese system of government at this time.

2 Was geographical isolation the only reason the Chinese did not have contact with the West? Give reasons for your answer.

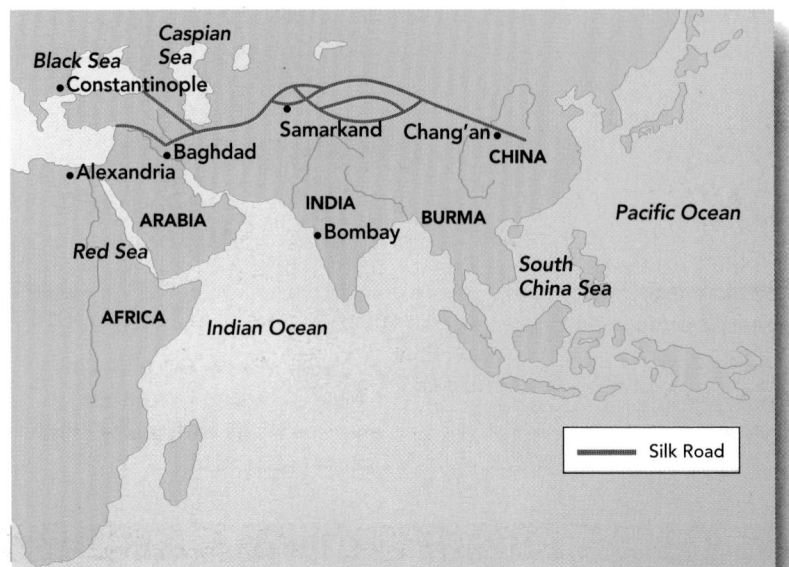

◄ The Silk Road showing the geographical isolation of China. All the goods carried along the Silk Road were carried by camels. The importance of camels is shown by the hundreds of pottery models of them in the tombs of emperors and nobles.

Chinese medicine is an energetic medicine whereas modern Western medicine is a biochemical medicine. Many of the medicinal traditions of the world are energetic rather than biochemical. An energetic medical tradition looks at the balance of the life force, humours or energy in the body, rather than at chemical reactions and its mechanical workings. All types of medicine study the same body. They just use different mental maps or theories of how the body works to decide what is happening.

Yin and Yang

One of the maps that the Chinese have based their medicine on for thousands of years is the principle of Yin and Yang – two opposing yet complementary forces.

Yin = cool, night, passive, inward, shade, rest. Yang = hot, day, active, outward, sun.	Yang 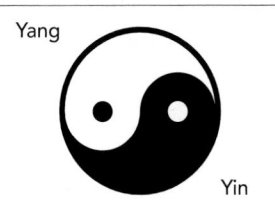 Yin

Ourselves and everything around us in the world are a balance of Yin and Yang. If a person is active all the time without rest, he or she will become ill. If the sun shines all day and night, the planet will burn up. The aim of Chinese medicine was to keep a balance between Yin and Yang in the body. To do this a doctor advised about diet and exercise and used herbs, acupuncture and moxibustion to restore the health of someone who had become ill.

Acupuncture and moxibustion

Acupuncture is the practice of inserting fine needles at certain points in the body to balance the energy or *qi* (pronounced chi in Chinese). This *qi* flows round the body in invisible channels. It can become blocked in some way and the needles can be used to restore the flow so that Yin and Yang can be in balance. Moxibustion is burning cones of a dried herb on the acupuncture points on the body to warm the *qi*.

Source H

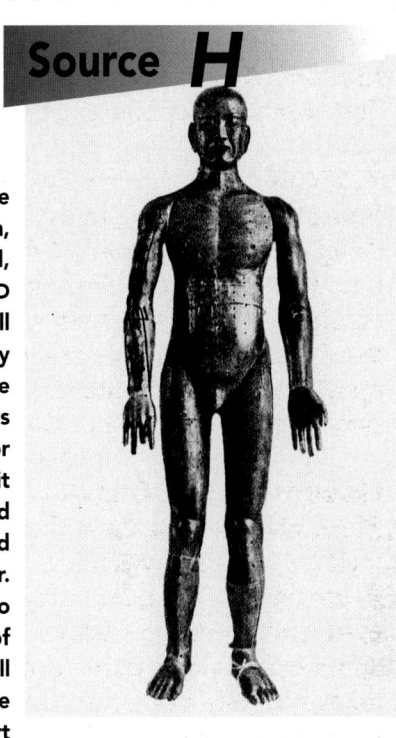

▶ The first life sized bronze man, so far discovered, was cast in AD 1027. It shows all the commonly used acupuncture points as pinholes. For examinations it could be covered with wax and filled with water. Students had to know the place of the points so well they could locate them and insert needles into them. If they were right, the water spurted out. This figure, only 26.2 centimetres high, was made by order of the emperor in 1726.

The earliest book on this subject is the *Huang Ti Nei Ching* (probably written about 100 BC). Since then some 30,000 volumes have been written about health and the treatment of disease using acupuncture, moxibustion and herbs. Chinese herbs have been widely used for centuries. Some Chinese doctors specialized in herbs alone, some in acupuncture. Most doctors, however, combined the two.

QUESTIONS

1 What steps might a Chinese doctor have taken to make someone well again?

2 a What similarities are there between Chinese medicine and Egyptian and Greek medicine?

b Can you explain these similarities?

CHAPTER 8

MEDICINE IN THE MIDDLE AGES

8.1 Western Europe in the Middle Ages

After the fall of the Roman Empire, Western Europe broke up into many small states. The only thing that unified it was religion. All the rulers would have accepted that they were part of **Christendom**. Only people in the Church, the educated (usually the same people) and some of the upper class would have read or understood Latin. It was for them an international language.

Compared with the 400 years after the fall of the Roman Empire, the Middle Ages were a period of growing peace. Larger countries were developing, like England, and, most of the time, they could maintain the rule of law at home. Little that was Roman had survived. The growing power of **Islam**, particularly in the Middle East slowly became a threat to Christendom and, from 1096 onwards, the **Crusades** brought the two cultures into fierce conflict.

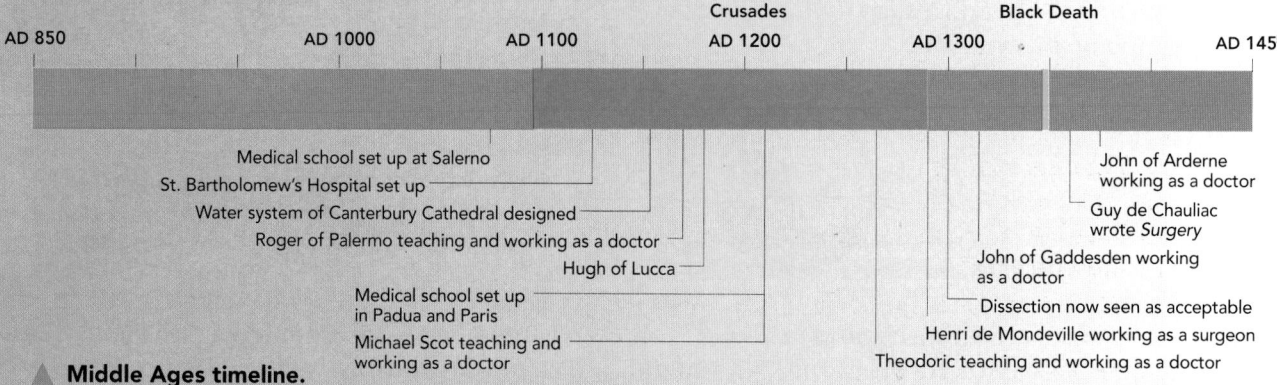

▲ **Middle Ages timeline.**

8.2 Beliefs about the causes of disease

Medieval people believed in a variety of different causes of disease. We can group many together and call them magical or supernatural. Others were physical. There were many different people to go to for diagnosis and treatment. There were doctors (usually very expensive), monks from the local monastery, apothecaries (people who sold herbs and drugs) and local wise men and women. There was not a simple link between the type of person you saw and the theory about disease. Doctors could prescribe charms, while many monks diagnosed and treated according to the theory of the four humours, as well as giving simple herbal remedies.

Source A

I permitted only red things to be about his bed, by which I cured him, without leaving a trace of the smallpox pustules on him.

▲ **From an account written by John of Gaddesden, the royal doctor at Edward II's court, in 1314. He is describing how he had cured Edward's son of smallpox by using *sympathetic* magic.**

Source B

For scrofula tumours and boils, use the herb scelerata softened and mixed with pig dung into a dough; apply to the scrofula tumours and boils and within a few hours it will waste them and the pus will disappear.

◀ From a 13th century medical manuscript. Scrofula was a disfiguring form of tuberculosis.

Source C

When scrofula comes to a head cut so that the pus comes out. If they harden and swell for a month or six months, or if the patient is a boy use this oil. At the declining of the moon make eleven poultices of iris and soft radish, use one every day from the tenth day on. Bleed the patient at least once in this period. If all this is not sufficient, surgery must be resorted to. The patient's throat should be firmly held with one hand while the outer skin is cut, then scraped and the scrofula caught with a hook and drawn out.

▲ From the 14th century writings of the doctor, Roger of Salerno.

The Church taught that God could send disease and misfortune as a punishment or as a test of faith, so prayer or a **pilgrimage** to a place like Canterbury, where saints were believed to perform miracle cures, were often thought to be a good idea. This was especially true for people who had diseases that could not be cured in any other way. The planets were also held to be responsible for disease, so medieval doctors were expected to have a good knowledge of **astrology** and **astronomy**. They needed to be able to chart the progress of the planets in the sky. This ability was seen as being just as important in diagnosing illness, as examining a patient, maybe more so.

There were also physical or natural theories about the cause of disease. The theory of the four humours was accepted by most of the better trained doctors. Urine analysis also played an important role in diagnosis. However, seemingly physical treatments, like herbal cures, could often be given for their supposed magical properties (herbs with a bitter taste, for example, were believed to drive away evil spirits), rather than for their actual scientific ones. Many doctors used a *Vademecum* to diagnose illness. This was a book that had the tables of the planets, a urine chart, and a set of rules for bleeding patients.

Source D

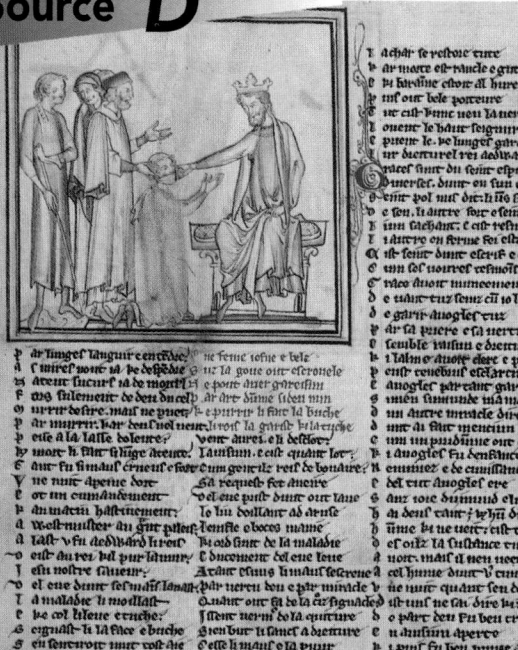

◀ In this illustration from a 13th century manuscript, Edward the Confessor touches a man to cure him from scrofula. Many kings and queens of England were believed to have the power to cure this disease, known as the 'King's Evil', by touch.

QUESTIONS

1 a Make a list of the different beliefs about causes of disease in the Middle Ages.

   b For each belief on your list explain why you think it was an old or a new idea.

2 What theory about the causes of disease lies behind the treatment in:

   a Source D

   b Source C?

   Give reasons for your answers.

The Middle Ages was a time of change in medicine, though this change was rather slow. The education and training of doctors was one of the first things to change.

Around the late 11th century, the first medical school of the period was set up at Salerno, in southern Italy. There is some evidence that this school produced women doctors as well as men, although it is not clear if these women doctors were supposed just to treat other women, especially during childbirth. The students worked with translations of the works of Galen and Hippocrates, and these translations were later used in other medical schools. Many of the works by Greek and Roman doctors had been saved only because they had been translated into Arabic. These were often translated back into Latin from Arabic. The rediscovery of the works of the ancients, and the discovery of the works of the Arabs was useful in many ways.

- The idea of clinical observation of the patient was stressed.
- The idea that cleanliness affected health gained a wider acceptance.
- The theory of the four humours and balance in the body was also revived.

Less useful was the fact that, for many teachers in the medical schools, what was in the books became 'the truth'. They taught students to believe everything written in the books, sometimes despite clear physical evidence to the contrary.

The medical school at Salerno became so influencial and well known that, in 1221, the Holy Roman Emperor Frederick made a law that only doctors who were approved at Salerno could practise medicine. This was an important step forward, although it applied only to the doctors who treated the rich and powerful, and it took many years for the practice of licensing doctors to be adopted by all countries. Gradually other medical schools were started. First Montpellier (12th century), then Bologna, Padua and Paris (13th century). With more schools, the number of trained doctors increased, as did the number of teachers and researchers. By the 14th century, there were many universities in Europe where students could train to become doctors. They were even allowed to witness dissection and take part in debates challenging the ideas of Galen and Hippocrates. It was largely as a result of these debates that some of the ideas that had been accepted for years were revised. New ideas, such as using urine colour as an aid to diagnosis, were developed as a result of close observation of the progress of diseases.

Source E

When you are asked if a sick person will escape from, or die of, his present illness, look at the ascendant [star sign] and where its lord is, since both signify the patient and his condition. Also examine the moon for the patient, because it is a witness of the fortune of this sick man concerning whom the question is made. Afterwards see the tenth house and its lord, since by them are signified health and medicine, or the virtue of the medicines and the advice of the physician. Then look at the sixth house and its lord, by whom the illness is denoted. Then see the eighth and its lord, by whom death for the sick is noted. Then see the fourth house and its lord, by whom the end for each of the aforesaid things is truly indicated.

▲ From the *Liber Introductorius*, written by Michael Scot. Scot was born around 1175 and was one of the most famous teachers and scholars at the medical school in Salerno.

Slow acceptance of new ideas

Not everyone accepted either the new ideas or the revisions to the old authorities. The ideas of Hippocrates and Galen still formed the basis of the textbooks that student doctors were taught from. Also, while ideas were debated, the debates were not always resolved in favour of the new ideas. They tended to be judged on the debating skills of the debaters, not on the medical evidence provided to support the claims of both sides.

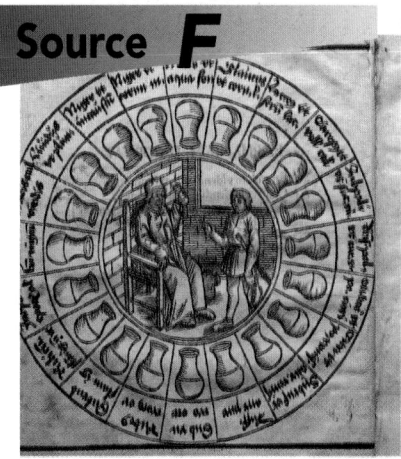

Source **F**

▲ A urine chart. This one comes from 1506, but they were in use much earlier than this. The use of the colour of urine to diagnose disease was one of the new ideas that became widely accepted.

8.4 Ordinary people

The developments described above were important, but did not have the same impact on everyone. While we know about the doctors who treated rich and powerful people, like popes and kings, we do not know how much these changes in thinking affected the treatment of ordinary people. The medical profession had a group of university-trained doctors at the top, treating the upper classes, who had very little in common with most people who practised medicine.

The changes in ideas had least effect in the countryside miles from the universities, where villagers went on treating diseases in the same way as they had done for centuries. For minor ailments, many people relied on cures passed down in their family that were known to work, or that were suggested by friends. They relied on local people, men and women, who had learned healing as a practical craft and had a reputation for successful magical or herbal cures. These people cared for the sick throughout the Middle Ages, but very few records of them or their activities have survived.

As towns grew, they attracted doctors. Doctors' fees were high. Many people could not afford a doctor when they were sick. Townspeople could ask the local apothecary (who sold herbs and drugs and sometimes charms) to suggest a cure. But they would have to pay for the drugs he suggested, even if the advice was free. Medical care, even at this level, was becoming specialized and beginning to exclude women. There were surgeons, **barber-surgeons** and doctors of physic. Women tended to act specifically as midwives. Some of these people had their skills passed on to them informally; others became apprentices and had a more formal training which ended in joining a guild.

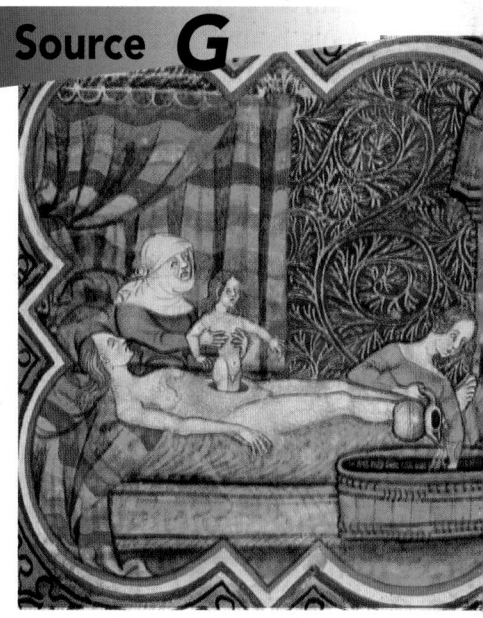

Source **G**

▲ A woman delivering a baby by *Caesarean section*. Women were eased out of medical practice until the only areas in which they were accepted were midwifery and as healers in the countryside.

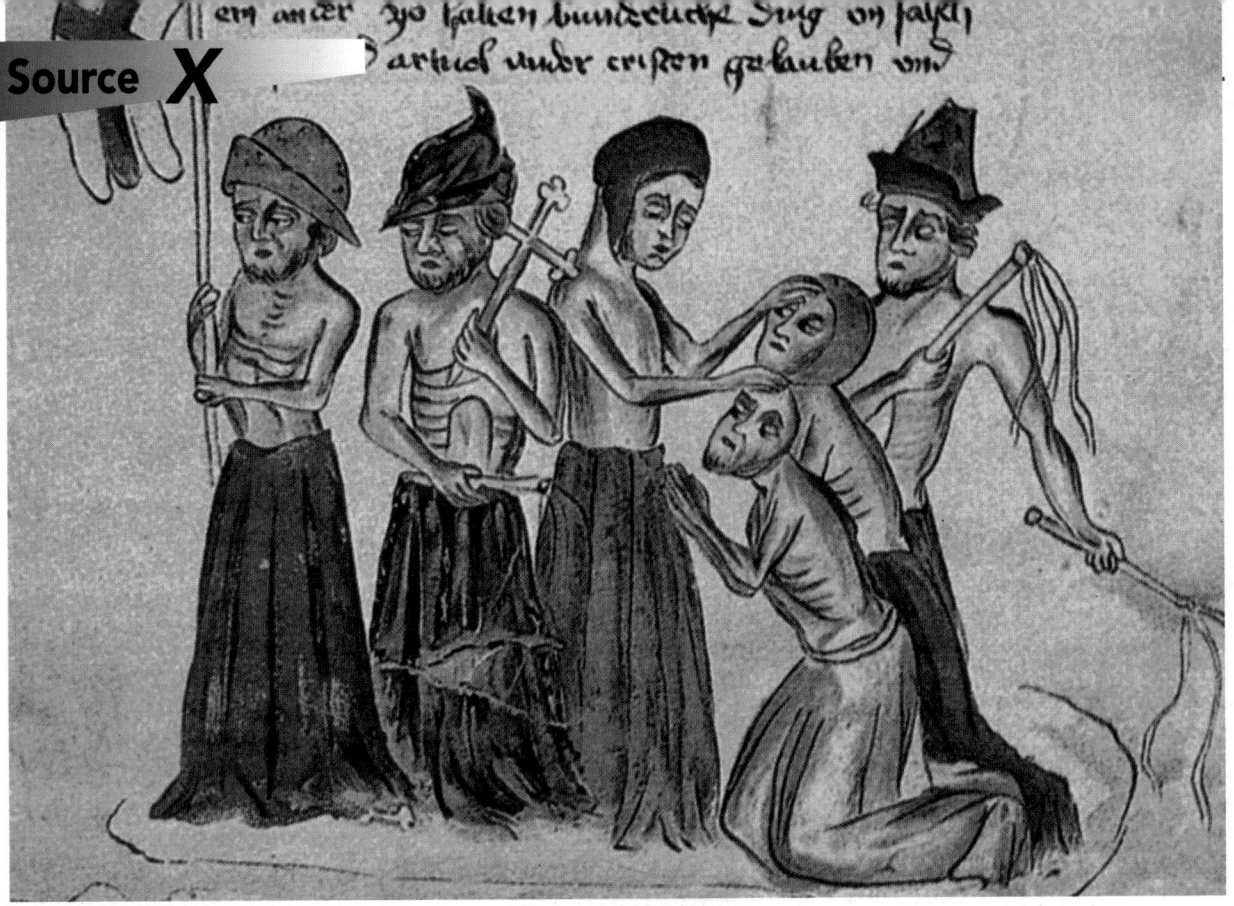

▲ Flagellants whipping themselves. These people thought the Black Death was sent by God because people were sinful. By punishing themselves they hoped God would be more merciful.

Source Y

About Michaelmas 1349, over six hundred men came to London from Flanders. Sometimes at St Paul's, and sometimes at other points in the city, they made two daily public appearances wearing clothes from the thighs to the ankle, but otherwise stripped bare. Each wore a cap with a red cross in front and behind. Each had in his right hand a scourge with three tails. Each tail had a knot and through the middle of it there were sometimes sharp nails fixed. They marched naked in a file one behind the other and whipped themselves with these scourges on their naked and bleeding bodies. Four of them would chant in their native tongues, and four would chant in response. Three times they would all cast themselves on the ground in this sort of procession, stretching out their hands like the arms of the cross. The singing would go on and on and each of them in turn would step over the others and give one stroke with his scourge to the man lying under him. This went on from the first to the last until each of them had observed the ritual.

▲ A description of the flagellants in London by a witness, the chronicler Robert of Avesbury.

QUESTIONS

1   Study Sources X and Y.

   a In what ways do the two sources support one another?

   b Are there any ways in which the sources contradict one another?

   c Both sources describe a fairly strange happening. Do you think they are reliable?

2   a What ways were suggested for preventing or curing the plague?

   b 'As people in the Middle Ages did not know what caused the plague none of their treatments can have been any good.' Explain why you agree or disagree with this statement.

8.8 Exercise

Study the following sources.

Source 1

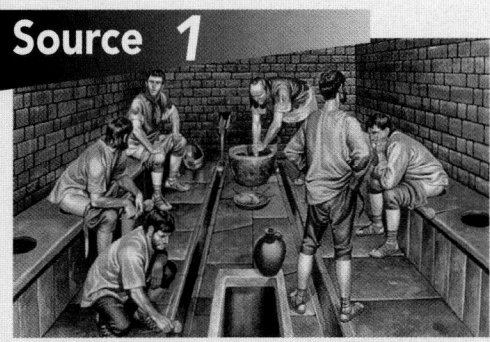

◀ A modern artist's reconstruction of a Roman lavatory on Hadrian's Wall. (See Source G on page 33.)

Source 2

▲ A plan of the water system of Canterbury Cathedral, 1153. (See Source M on page 54.)

Source 3

The lane called Ebbegate which runs between the tenements of Master John de Pulteneye and Master Thomas at Wytte used to be a right of way to all men until it was closed up by Thomas at Wytte and William de Hockele who got together and built latrines which stuck out from the walls of the houses. From these latrines human filth falls out onto the heads of passers-by.

▲ Evidence given in a court case heard in London, in 1321.

1 Why were the sewage disposal systems in Source 3 so different from those in Source 1?

2 Why were the sewage disposal systems in Source 3 so different to those in Source 2?

3 Does Source 3 show people had stopped thinking hygiene was important?

Copy and complete the summary chart below.

Medicine in the Middle Ages					
Factors affecting Medicine		Causes of Disease		New Features	
Factor	Effect	Cause	Evidence	Feature	Evidence
1 _____	Survival of some Greek and Roman medical books.	1 Supernatural	a) _____ b) _____ c) _____	1 Use of wine as a simple antiseptic.	_____
		2 Physical	a) Bad air b) _____ c) _____	2 Use of opium as an anaesthetic.	
		Treatments Used		3 Formal training for doctors at Medical Schools and Universities.	a) Salerno (11th century) b) Montpellier (12th century) c) _____
		Treatment	Illness	Evidence	
		1 Pilgrimage	_____	shrines and offerings	
		2 Poultices, bleeding and surgery	_____	Roger of Salerno (Source C)	
2 _____	Trade with the Arabs meant: a) Works by Galen and other Classical authors returned to the West. b) New ideas from Islamic doctors.	3 Sympathetic magic	_____	John of Gaddesden	4 Books for doctors to carry round with them and use to help in diagnosis.	_____
		4 Royal touch	_____	C13 Manuscript (Source D)	
		5 Herbs mixed with pig dung.	_____	C13 Manuscript (Source B)	
		6 Cleaning towns to remove rubbish and sewage.	_____	Order from Edward III to the Lord Mayor of London. (Source U)	5 _____	Urine charts
		7 People punishing themselves so God would forgive sins.	The plague	_____		

CHAPTER 9

MEDICINE IN EARLY MODERN EUROPE

9.1 Renaissance and Reformation

The Middle Ages had been a period of slow change. Between 1430 and 1700 (usually called the Early Modern period by historians) Europe was in a ferment of change. Old ideas were being challenged. New ideas were proclaimed and challenged in their turn.

Renaissance means re-birth. It describes the new interest in the culture and science of the Greeks and Romans. Scholars started by going back to the original Greek or Latin texts, many of which were made available for the first time. Scholars not only read the texts but also began to adopt the enquiring attitudes of the classical authors. They accepted the importance of the close observation of nature and the need to make theories which explained the world. A movement which began by looking backwards finished by looking forwards.

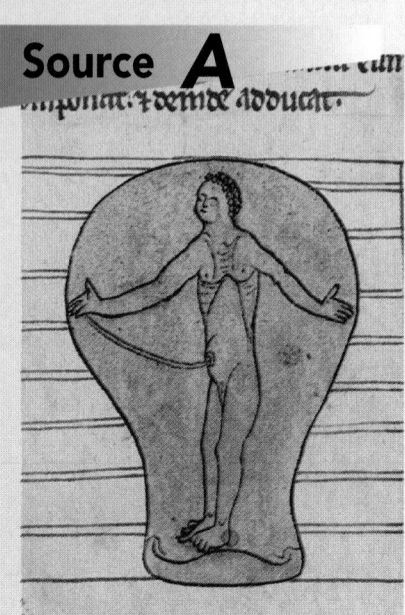

◀ A drawing of a foetus from a medieval book for midwives.

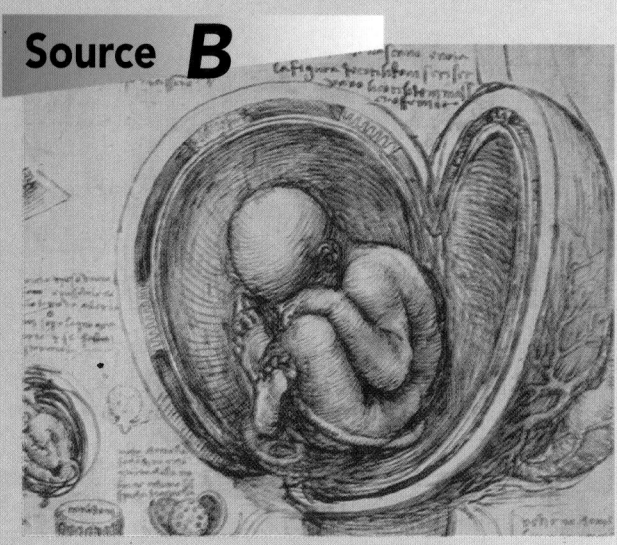

▲ A drawing of a foetus by Leonardo da Vinci. He was able to dissect the body of a woman who died during pregnancy before making the drawing.

There were important developments in art during the Renaissance. The great artists insisted that art had to be based on the most accurate observation possible. Artists attended human dissections so that they understood the structure of the body and were better able to paint it. This, in turn, helped medicine. The artists who worked with anatomists were able to bring a new realism to their work.

The Reformation was an equally dramatic change, this time in religious beliefs and practices. Again it started by looking backwards. People thinking about how the Church should be organized thought the early Church in the years immediately after the death of Christ must be the best blueprint and that later changes should be swept away. The Pope, who was one of the later changes, did not agree.

Printing

There were important changes in technology as well. Johann Gutenberg introduced printing into Europe in 1454. As you can see from the map, printing spread very quickly. Its effects were enormous. Books were the best way to spread knowledge and ideas. Before Gutenberg, making a book, especially an illustrated one, had been a very labour intensive process. Each picture had to be copied again. Think of the value of illustrations in a book on anatomy. It is not surprising there were very few copies of most books around before printing and that the illustrations in medical books were often poor. A combination of the skill of the artists and the time taken by the copyists meant medical books had been illustrated by drawings such as Source A. Printing and the new skills of the artists meant in future they would look more like Source F on page 63.

This ferment of ideas affected medicine. The changes in attitude happened gradually over half-a-century, but the events of one month, in 1527, sum them all up. Paracelsus was appointed town physician and lecturer to the university in Basel. He nailed an invitation to all people, including barber-surgeons, not just students, to the door of his lecture theatre. Three weeks later he started his first lecture by burning books by Galen and Avicenna. He then lectured in German, the language of the region, not Latin. He went on to say, *'Galen is a liar and a fake. Avicenna is a kitchen master. They are good for nothing. You will not need them. Reading never made a doctor. Patients are the only books. You will follow me.'*

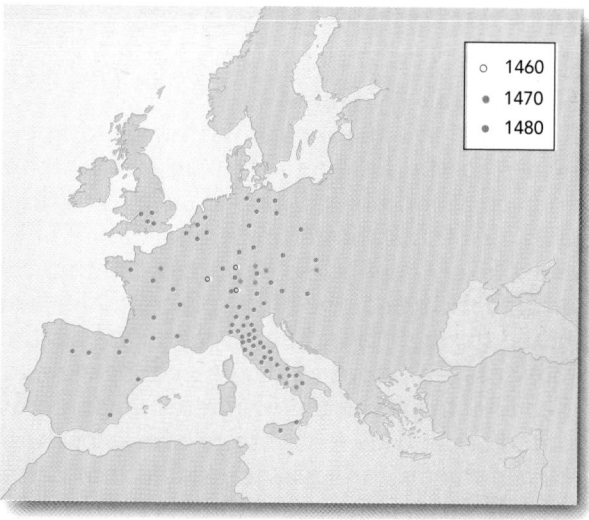

▲ **The spread of printers' workshops 1460-80.**

QUESTIONS

1 What effect could changes in art have on medicine?

2 'Medicine has often been affected by changes in technology that are not changes in medical technology.' Can this be true? Explain your answer.

3 Within a year of his first lecture, Paracelsus had been forced to flee from Basel at the dead of night in fear of his life. Does this mean his lecture cannot have been important in the development of medicine? Explain your answer.

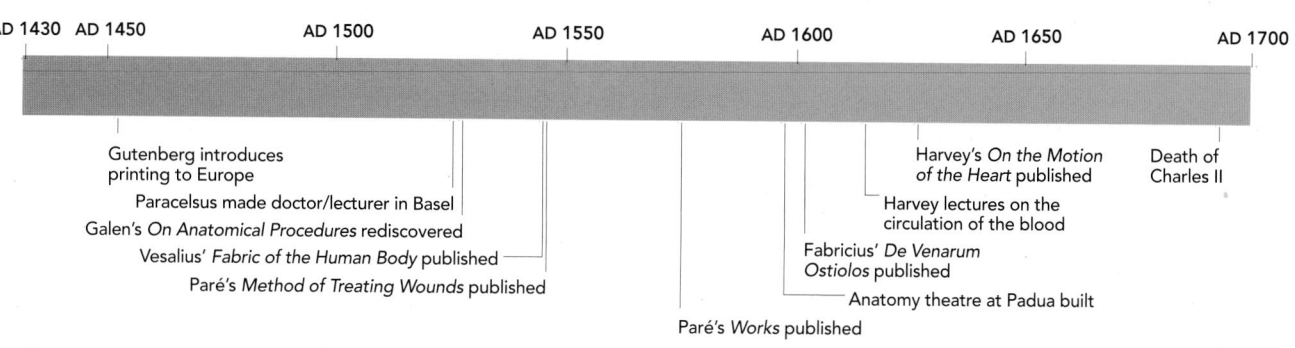

▲ **Early Modern medicine 1430–1700.**

A new book by Galen

Most of Galen's anatomical writings had not been available during the Middle Ages. The standard textbook on anatomy had been Mondino de Luzzi's *Anatomy*, written in 1316, and based on a translation from Arabic of half of *On the Use of the Parts*, one of Galen's less important anatomical books. Through the rest of the Middle Ages Galen's anatomy was studied through Mondino's version. It was this book that professors read from while dissections were taking place. After 1500 there was a new interest in anatomy. People wanted to get back to the 'pure' works of the classical masters. *On the use of the Parts* was translated into Latin and published in full. In 1531, Johannes Guinter, Professor of Medicine at Paris, published a Latin translation of Galen's *On Anatomical Procedures*, his major work on anatomy – lost in the West since the fall of the Roman Empire. This lost book transformed the study of anatomy. It was vastly superior to Mondino's. Galen insisted the study of anatomy started with the skeleton. He regretted not being able to use human dissection as the basis for his work, insisting it was necessary. His system for the study of anatomy was quite different from Mondino's. It was adopted without reservation throughout the West.

Vesalius' early life

Andreas Vesalius was born into a medical family. His father was apothecary to the Holy Roman Emperor Charles V and his grandfather, great-grandfather, and great-great-grandfather had all been doctors. Born in Brussels in 1514, he grew up in a house with medical books. He studied at the university in Louvain between 1528 and 1533, when he moved on to Paris. There he began to study medicine and attracted attention as a good anatomist. In 1536 he had to leave because war broke out between the Emperor Charles V and France. He returned to Louvain where he continued to study anatomy. Human dissection had been allowed throughout the Middle Ages, but boiling up bodies to produce skeletons had been forbidden since 1300. While at Louvain, Vesalius went to great lengths to get a skeleton. He went to a gibbet outside the town where executed criminals were displayed. *'I happened upon a dried cadaver. The bones were entirely bare, held together by the ligaments alone. . . . I climbed the stake and pulled off the femur from the hip bone. While tugging at the specimen, the shoulder blades together with the arms and hands also followed... After I had brought the legs and arms home in secret and successive trips (leaving the head behind with the entire trunk of the body), I allowed myself to be shut out of the city in the evening in order to obtain the trunk, which was firmly held by a chain. The next day I transported the bones home piecemeal through another gate of the city.'*

Source C

As poles to tents, and walls to houses, so are bones to living creatures, for other features naturally take form from them and change with them.

▲ From *On Anatomical Procedures*, written by Galen in about AD 200 but lost, after the fall of Rome, until 1531.

Source D

I would not mind having as many cuts inflicted on me as I have seen him make either on man or other animal [except at the banqueting table].

▲ Vesalius on Johannes Guinter. He is implying that Guinter did not do any dissecting.

Source E

As the gods love me, I, who yield to none in my devotion and reverence to Galen, neither can nor should enjoy any greater pleasure than praising him.

▲ Vesalius, in answer to criticism that he was unrestrained in his criticisms of Galen.

Vesalius at Padua

Vesalius did not stay in Louvain long. He fell out with the professor of medicine over the correct way to bleed patients. He left in 1537 and went to Padua in Italy. Although still a young man, he was appointed professor of surgery. In Padua the professor of surgery was also responsible for teaching anatomy. The next five years in Padua were the most creative of Vesalius' life.

He taught anatomy, breaking with tradition by doing his own dissections, and then by publishing drawings. Many doctors at the time argued that drawings had no place in proper science. Vesalius disagreed. He felt that drawings of various parts of the body would help students watching a dissection, and help them learn about the body before and after dissections. In 1538 he published his *Tabulae Sex*, six large sheets of anatomical drawings. Source F shows one of these sheets. Imagine trying to describe what is shown in words, without the use of pictures or diagrams.

The *Tabulae Sex* showed that Vesalius was starting to see some of the problems in Galen's anatomy, but that he was not yet ready to reject Galen's theories openly. In Source F he shows a five-lobed liver, as described by Galen, but as found in animals not humans. In the first sheet, he shows two more views of the liver. The main one shows the five-lobed liver again, but the smaller view shows a two-lobed liver of the sort found in humans rather than animals.

In 1539 Vesalius published his *Letter on Venesection*. Venesection was the practice of bleeding patients. The medical books of the Middle Ages, following the work of the Arab doctors, said the vein to be opened should be on the opposite side of the body from the site of the illness, and that only a small amount of blood should be taken. This theory was criticized by those doctors who wanted to get back to the 'pure' medicine of Hippocrates and Galen. Hippocrates and Galen had not said bleeding should happen on the opposite side of the body, and had suggested taking more blood. This was the argument which got Vesalius in trouble with the professor in Louvain. Vesalius was on the side of the purists. Other books in this controversy had argued on the basis of what Galen and Hippocrates had actually written, or that certain patients had got better when bled in one way or the other. Vesalius put the argument on a much more scientific basis. He showed, again through illustrations, how the veins were connected. He provided an anatomical reason to accept the theories of Galen and Hippocrates.

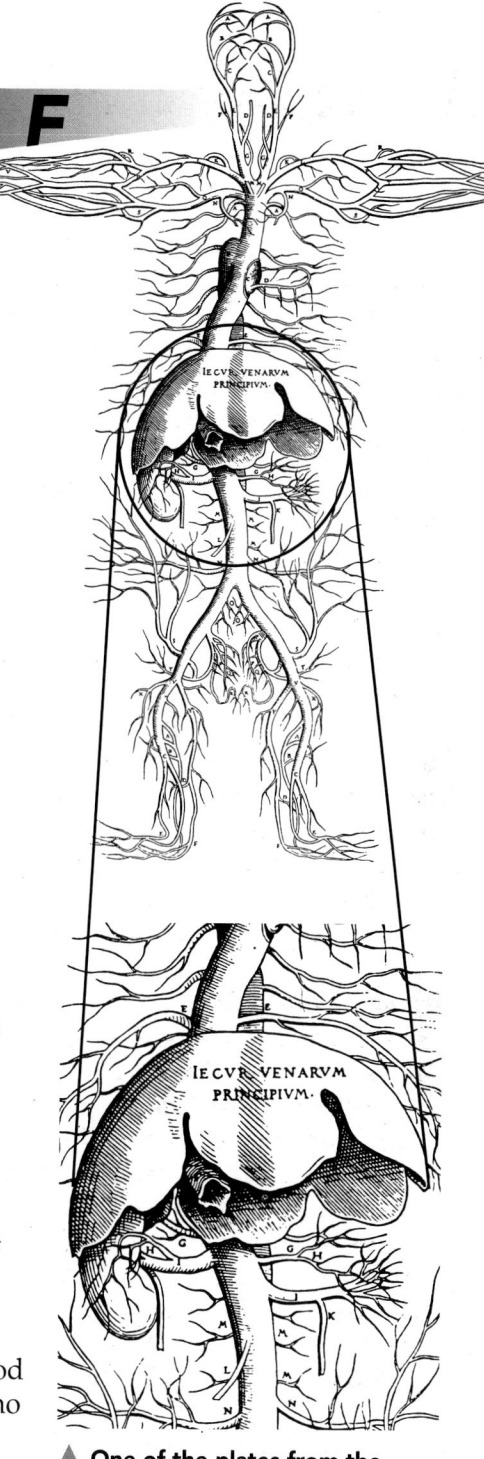

Source F

▲ One of the plates from the *Tabulae Sex*, Vesalius' first major work on anatomy, published in 1538. This plate was engraved from one of Vesalius' own drawings. It shows the ideas of Galen. The liver (see detail) is shown as a five lobed organ as Galen described it. This is the shape of an animal liver, not a human liver, which has only two lobes.

The Fabric of the Human Body 1543

Vesalius spent his time in Padua working on his great book, *The Fabric of the Human Body*. It was a comprehensive study of human anatomy, illustrated throughout by the work of first-class artists from the studio of Titian, one of the great painters of the Renaissance. Its publication was one of the great moments in the history of medicine.

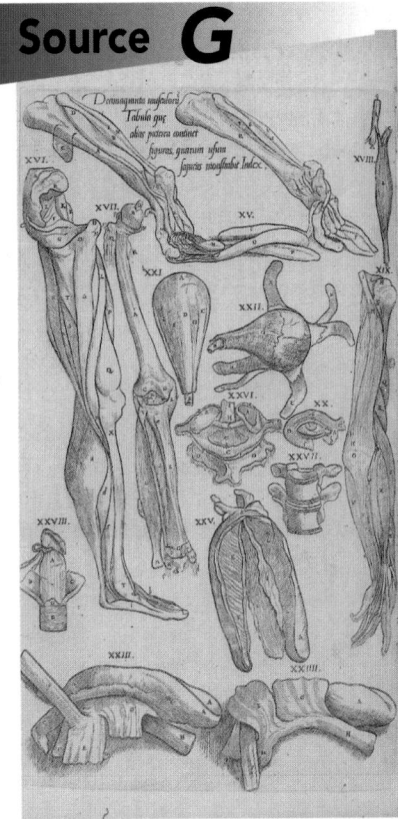

▲ The 16th plate from Vesalius' description of the muscles. Notice the letters and numbers so the parts can be named and keyed into Vesalius' text.

- It offered a complete human anatomy based on a comprehensive programme of human dissection. Within each section Vesalius starts from the most complete picture and works down from this. Thus the section on muscles starts with a flayed body displaying all the surface muscle groups, and ends, after each layer of muscles is removed in turn, with a few individual muscles.
- It corrected some errors in Galen's anatomy.
- It offered a method by which the study of anatomy could progress – public dissection and the publication of work backed up with illustrations.
- It broke new ground in the relationship between the illustrations and the text. All Vesalius' illustrations have letters on them. These letters were not just used to key in a list of the names of the parts. Vesalius constantly referred to the letters in his text, making the book one where the pictures and text were integrated into one complete explanation.
- Vesalius painstakingly oversaw the preparation of the wood-block engravings that were used to print the illustrations and every stage in the publication of his work. In 1543 he left Padua to spend months with the printer in Basel so that everything was checked and correct. Because Vesalius' theories were in printed-book form there was no shortage of copies. These were quickly distributed around the great centres of learning in Europe and other anatomists could judge Vesalius' work for themselves, studying the text and illustrations in their own time.

The Fabric of the Human Body was not the only book Vesalius published in 1543. At the same time, he produced the *Epitome*. This was a small summary of *The Fabric*. The publication of *The Fabric* and the *Epitome* did not, however, change the study of anatomy overnight. Many of the other anatomists of the day, whose work was challenged and refuted by Vesalius, put up a strong fight. However, Vesalius' method – dissection and illustration – was difficult to argue with.

Vesalius' later life

Vesalius dedicated *The Fabric* to the Holy Roman Emperor Charles V. He hoped for, and was given, a job at Charles' court. A second edition of *The Fabric*, published in 1555, added a number of new observations, but Vesalius worked on as a doctor not an anatomist. He left the court in 1564, intending to return to Padua and teaching. However, he died before he could return.

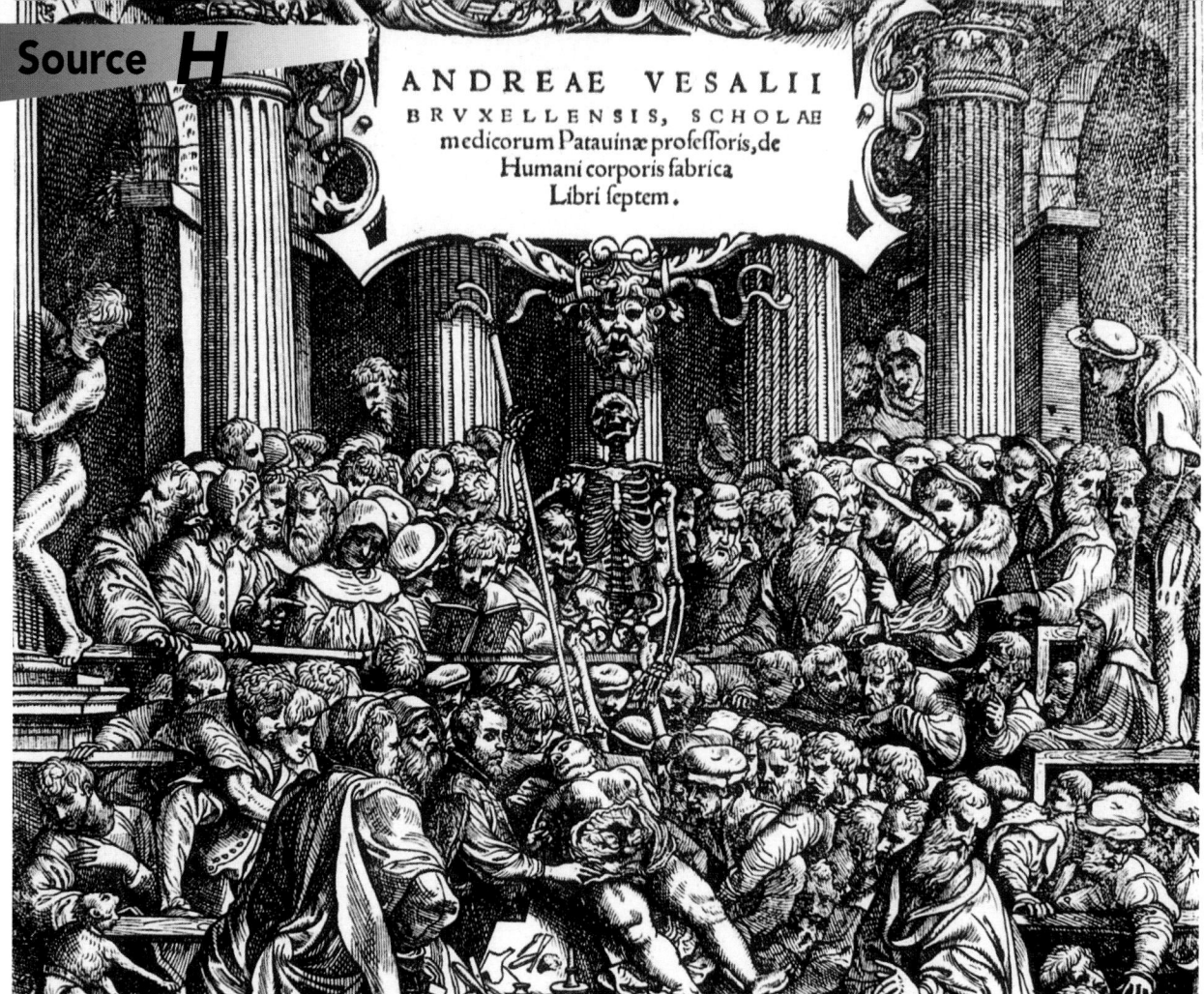

ANDREAE VESALII
BRVXELLENSIS, SCHOLAE
medicorum Patauinæ profefforis, de
Humani corporis fabrica
Libri feptem.

▲ The title page of the 1543 edition of *The Fabric of the Human Body.* Vesalius is shown doing the dissection, which is taking place outdoors. This was common at the time, and temporary wooden stands were built to enable as many as possible to watch the dissection.

TRENDS AND TURNING POINTS

A **trend** takes place over a long time. It is a gradual change made up of a series of events.

A **turning point** is something that happens quickly and it may be just one event. Afterwards, things are different in at least one important way.

QUESTIONS

1 'Galen was the first of the new anatomists of the 16th century'. Can this statement be true?

2 Explain the importance of:

  a the *Tabulae Sex*
  b the *Letter on Venesection*
  c *The Fabric of the Human Body.*

3 Vesalius was able to correct errors in people's ideas about the human body that had lasted for centuries. Why did some people object to his work?

4 Improvements in drawing and the development of printing are often said to be part of the reason for Vesalius' success.

  a How did these developments help Vesalius?
  b Are these developments, by themselves, enough to explain why Vesalius was so successful?

5 Was the publication of *The Fabric of the Human Body* a turning point, or part of a trend in the history of medicine?

Paré, the son of a barber-surgeon, was born in a small village in France in 1510. Barber-surgeons were the lowest of the low in 16th century French medicine. When Paré died, aged 80, however, he had been surgeon to four successive kings of France, and he was the most famous surgeon of his age.

Paré went to Paris to train as a barber-surgeon in 1533. In 1534 he became the surgeon to the *Hôtel-Dieu* which was the only public hospital in Paris. In 1537 he left and joined the French army as a military surgeon, perhaps because he did not have enough money to take the examinations to qualify as a barber-surgeon. He was a very successful military surgeon and, as France was often either at war or engaged in civil war, there was plenty of opportunity to practise his craft. The musket was becoming the most important weapon on the battlefield and Paré developed a new way of treating gunshot wounds. In 1545 he published his first book on the treatment of gunshot wounds, *Method of Treating Wounds*. It was written in French not Latin, the usual language of medical books, as Paré did not speak Latin.

In 1552 Paré was appointed surgeon to Henri II of France and continued to develop new treatments, and to publish books about them. The first edition of his collected works was published in 1575. This led to an attack on him by the Faculty of Physicians, the people at the top of France's medical tree. Étienne Gourmelen, Dean of the Faculty, said Paré was an ignorant charlatan and insisted no medical books could be published without the Faculty's approval. This was the law, but Paré had the king's support. Nothing was done to stop the sale of his works, and they went into three more editions during his lifetime. The attack did spur Paré to write his own life story, *The Apology and Treatise of Ambroise Paré*, which was published in 1585. Because Paré was such a determined author we can study some of his most important cases in his own words.

Source I

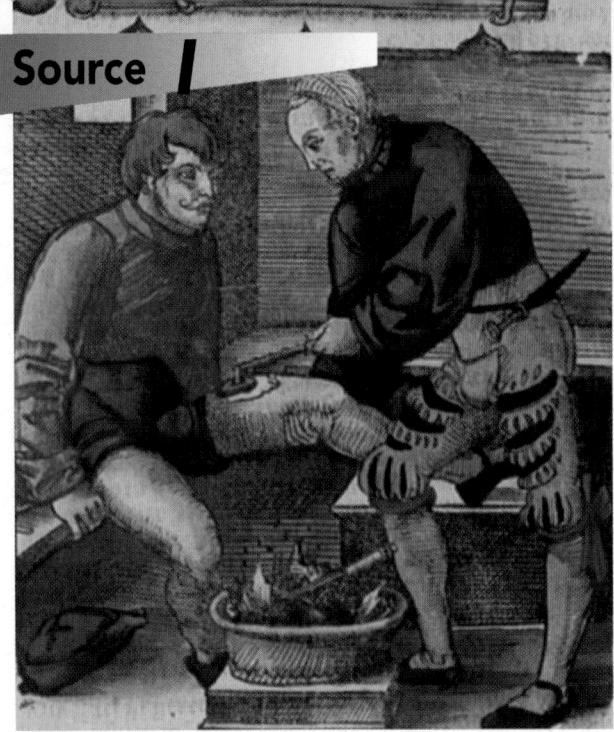

▲ The treatment of gunshot wounds before Paré. This print, from a manual for surgeons, shows the accepted treatment. Gunshot wounds were thought to be poisonous. They were either burnt with a red hot iron (called a *cautery*) or they were filled with boiling oil. People believed this would counteract the poison.

Source J

Dare you say you will teach me surgery, you who have never come out of your study? ... Surgery is learned by the eye and the hands. I can perform surgical operations which you cannot do, because you have never left your study or the schools. Diseases are not to be cured by eloquence, but by treatment well and truly applied. You, my little master, know nothing else but how to chatter in a chair.

[Later Paré describes the scene after the battle of St Quentin, when the ground was covered with so many dead men and horses and] ...so many blue and green flies rose from them they hid the sun; where they settled there they infested the air and brought the plague with them. My little master I wish you had been there.

▲ From the *Apology and Treatise of Ambroise Paré*, 1585, in which he refers to Gourmelen (my little master) who had criticized and tried to suppress his writings. 'My little master I wish you had been there' is a phrase which runs through the book.

Source K

Now at that time I was a fresh water soldier, I had not yet seen wounds made by gunpowder at the first dressing. I had read that wounds made with weapons of fire were poisoned, by reason of the powder, and they should be treated by cauterizing them with oil scalding hot, in which should be mingled a little treacle. Before I used this treatment, knowing it would cause the patient great pain, I wanted to know what the other surgeons did. They applied the oil, as hot as was possible, into the wounds. I took courage to do as they did.

Eventually I ran out of oil. I was forced instead to use an ointment made from yolks of eggs, oil of roses, and turpentine. That night I could not sleep, fearing what would happen because the wounds were not cauterized and that I should find those on whom I had not used the burning oil dead or poisoned. This made me rise up very early to visit them. To my surprise I found those to whom I gave my ointment feeling little pain, and their wounds without inflammation or swelling, having rested reasonably well during the night. Whereas the others, on whom I used the boiling oil, were feverish, with great pain and swelling about the edges of their wounds. And then I resolved with myself never so cruelly to burn poor men wounded with gunshot.

▲ An account of his discovery of his improved method for treating gunshot wounds, from *The Apology*, 1585. Paré had published an account of this method of treatment as early as 1545.

Source L

Where the amputation must be made

Let us suppose that the foot is mortified, even to the ankle. You must carefully mark in what place you must cut it off. You shall cut off as little that is sound as you possibly can.

How the amputation must be performed

The first care must be of the patient's strength. Let him be nourished with meats, yolks of eggs, and bread toasted and dipped in wine. Then let him be placed as is fit, and draw the muscles upwards toward the sound parts, and let them be tied with a ligature a little above the place which is to be cut. This ligature has three uses. First to hold the muscles and skin drawn up so that later they may cover the ends of the cut bones. Second to slow the flow of blood by pressing and shutting up the veins and arteries. Third it must dull the sense of the part. When you have made your ligature cut the flesh even to the bone with a sharp and well-cutting knife or with a crooked knife.

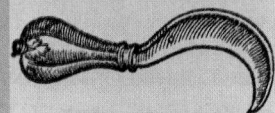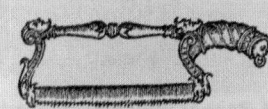

If you leave anything but bone to be cut by the saw you will put the patient to excessive pain. When you come to the bared bone cut it with a little saw, some foot and three inches long. Then you must smooth the front of the bone that the saw has made rough.

How to stop the bleeding

Let it bleed a little then let the veins and arteries be tied up as speedily as you can so that the course of the flowing blood may be stopped. This may be done by taking hold of the vessels with your Crow's Beak, which looks like this.

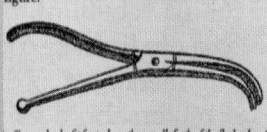

The ends of the vessels lying hidden in the flesh, must be drawn out with this instrument. When you have so drawn them forth bind them with double thread.

Formerly I used to stop the bleeding in another way, of which I am ashamed, but what should I do. I had observed my masters whose method I intended to follow, who used hot irons. This kind of treatment could not but bring great and tormenting pain to the patient. And truly of those that were burnt, the third part scarce recovered. I entreat all surgeons to leave this old and too cruel way of healing, and embrace this new.

▲ From *Of Amputations*, which appeared in Paré's *Works*, 1575.

THE DOCTOR – THOMAS SYDENHAM

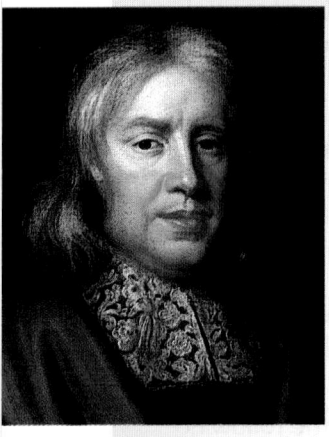

Sydenham was one of the most successful doctors in London from 1656 until his death in 1689. He has been called 'The English Hippocrates' because he stressed the importance of close observation of patients and their symptoms. His advice to a young man wanting to become a doctor was clear:

'Anatomy, botany – nonsense. Sir, I know an old woman in the flower market who understands botany better. As for anatomy, my butcher can dissect a joint just as well. No, young man, all this is stuff. You must go to the bedside. It is there alone you can learn about disease.'

Sydenham often thought the best treatment was to leave the patient alone so they could get over their own disease. Other treatments relied on common-sense. Roast chicken and a bottle of wine for a man weakened by repeated bleedings and purgings by other doctors. Hippocrates had done the same. Sydenham's close observation enabled him to discover a new disease. He was the first doctor to describe **scarlet fever**.

In a letter to a medical colleague Sydenham described his method:

'I have been very careful to write nothing but what was the product of faithful observation and neither suffered myself to be deceived by idle speculations nor have deceived others by obtruding anything upon them but downright matters of fact.'

WOMEN

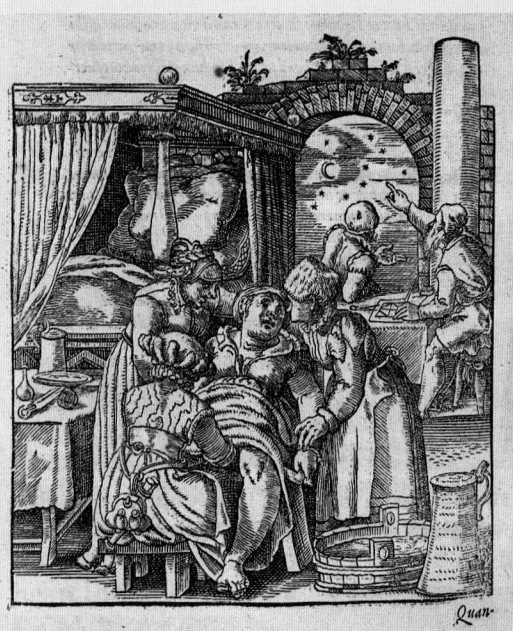

A woman giving birth. This illustration comes from a book printed in 1580, but the way things were done had not changed by the middle of the 17th century. The woman is being helped by a midwife and comforted by her friends. The two doctors are in the background casting the new-born baby's horoscope. Midwives were usually women. Some were just experienced older women who helped their neighbours. Most, though, were paid and had learnt the job by spending time with another midwife.

There were a few women surgeons and doctors in 17th century England, but they were becoming less common than they had been in the Middle Ages. Formal medicine, practised by qualified people, was becoming a male preserve. There were some professional nurses, usually women, but most nursing was done by the sick person's family or friends.

Many people did not go for treatment to a qualified doctor. There might not be one near to where they lived, or they might not be able to afford to visit one, or they just might not have liked the idea. They used informal healers – witches, wise-women or wizards, or even the lady of the manor all treated the sick. Women played an important part in most people's lives during illness. If you were sick in 1660, you might have been more likely to see a woman healer than a qualified male doctor.

DIFFERENT TYPES OF TREATMENT

If you are ill today you will probably be treated by a conventional doctor working within the tradition of western medicine. You could, however, find other sorts of treatment: acupuncture, faith healing, and homeopathy, for instance, are all practised in modern Britain. This range of different types of treatment was more common in the 17th century. Trained doctors and surgeons might very well have very different ideas about the cause of a disease and the type of treatment that would prove most suitable. Patients could also try magical and supernatural cures. When we read about people's illnesses in diaries and letters from the time we often see they used many kinds of treatments – often consulting more than one person in order to get a wide range of possible remedies. The trained doctors often wanted to stop other people working as healers. They often accused people like this of being untrained and dangerous. Some thought that this was because they wanted to keep all the fees to themselves. Many trained doctors believed in supernatural as well as natural cures. Here Robert Burton, a doctor, advises against using magical healers, not because their cures did not work, but because they did work. He thought the Devil might cure illness but trap the patient into witchcraft.

'Evil is not to be done that good may come of it. Much better it were for such patients, that are so troubled, to endure a little misery in this life, than to risk their soul's health forever, and much better to die than be so cured.'

QUESTIONS

1 Why were doctors not able to extend their scientific methods to treatment?

2 a How do you think the woman in the childbirth picture would have felt about the doctors studying the stars and ignoring her labour?

   b How might Sydenham have treated Charles II?

3 Robert Burton believed magical cures worked, but people should not use them. Why?

4 'The treatment of Charles II shows that doctors had rejected the work of Paré and Harvey.' Do you agree with this statement?

CHARLES II

Like many English kings since the Middle Ages, Charles 'touched' people to cure them of scrofula (see page 49 Source D). During his reign Charles touched 90,798 of his subjects to cure them.

In 1685 Charles was sick with what turned out to be his fatal illness. His doctors tried many treatments – remember, as you read them, that Charles was the king, the most important man in the country. He had the best doctors available. One of them, Sir Charles Scarburgh, left us an account of the treatment:

2 February *'The king ...felt some unusual disturbance in his brain, soon followed by loss of speech and convulsions. Two of the king's physicians ...opened a vein in his right arm, and drew off about 16 ounces [454 grams] of blood. Meantime, the rest of the Physicians had been summoned by express messengers... '*

The treatment continued:

Eight more ounces [227 grams] of blood let, then pills to *'drain away the humours'*, and medicine to make him vomit.

3 February Sacred Tincture every six hours [a laxative]. Ten ounces [280 grams] of blood were let from the jugular veins, after which the king complained of a sore throat.

4 February More laxative. Then, as Charles got worse, a medicine which included 40 drops of essence of human skull.

5 February Peruvian bark [quinine].

6 February *'As the illness was now becoming more grave and his Majesty's strength gradually failing'* a cardiac tonic was tried, then a medicine including bezoar stone. Charles died.

9.6 Exercise

Study the following sources.

Source 1

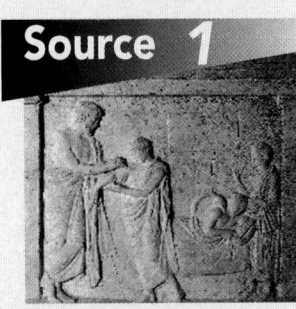

▲ Asclepios treating Archionos, 350 BC.

Source 2

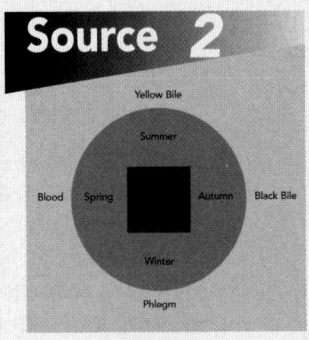

▲ The four humours.

Source 3

4 February 1685. The physicians considered it necessary to open both jugular veins and draw off about 10 ounces [280 ml] of blood.

▲ From Sir Charles Scarburgh's account of the death of Charles II.

You will find it helpful to look back at Source 1 on page 23 and Source 2 on page 25, where they are shown much larger.

1 What differences are there in the beliefs about the cause and cure of disease between Sources 1 and 2?

2 Source 3 is about 2,000 years later than Source 2, yet it shares the same beliefs about cause and cure of disease. How can this be explained?

3 Between 400 BC and 1685 some things in medicine changed and some stayed the same. Which was more important in the history of medicine between those dates, things which changed or things which stayed the same? Support your answer with reasons and examples.

4 The 200 years before 1685 are seen as very important in the development of medicine yet the treatment of Charles II was not very effective. Why?

Copy and complete the summary chart below.

Early Modern Medicine						
Factors affecting Medicine		**Causes of Disease**		**New Features**		
Factor	Effect	Cause	Evidence	Feature	Evidence	
1 Communications: a) development of printing b) accuracy of drawing	_____	Physical causes: The Four Humours, Supernatural causes	_____ _____	Improvements in anatomy: 1 Vesalius ensures anatomy based on human dissection, corrects many errors, and establishes need for illustration in anatomical books.	_____	

Treatments Used			
Treatment	Illness	Evidence	
1 Cautery	Gunshot wounds and amputations	_____	
2 Ointment and bandaging	Gunshot wounds	_____	
3 Ligature, and tying blood vessels with thread.	Amputations	_____	
4 _____	Any illness	Robert Burton	
5 Bleeding and purging	Illnesses with fever, swelling and/or convulsions	_____	

Factor	Effect
2 Technology: the invention of pumps to drain mines and fight fires.	_____
3 _____	Wounds treated led to new treatments being developed such as Paré's use of ligatures.
4 _____	Paré developed his new treatment for gunshot wounds because he ran out of boiling oil to use as a cautery.

Feature	Evidence
2 Function of the heart and circulation of the blood discovered.	
Improvements in surgery: use of ligatures in amputations.	_____
A more scientific attitude to proof – especially the growing use of experiments.	a) Vesalius' use of public dissection to prove his theories. b) c) Harvey's experiments described in *On the Motion of the Heart*, 1628.
Printed books made new ideas more widely available more quickly.	_____

MEDICINE ON THE BRINK

10.1 The old order begins to change

The interest in science and experimentation continued into the 18th century. Physics became more established. The microscope had been invented as early as 1683 by the Dutchman, Anthony van Leeuwenhoek. This was now followed by the thermometer, invented by Fahrenheit in 1709 and Celsius in 1742. In chemistry a number of new substances were discovered such as hydrogen, oxygen, and nitrous oxide. These inventions and discoveries, however, did not make an impact on medicine until the 19th century.

Nevertheless, it was a time when old ideas about medicine were questioned. Physicians, such as Hermann Boerhaave, were stimulated into observing patients more closely and keeping accurate records (see box). Boerhaave also caused a new edition of Vesalius' work to be published, as many doctors were keen to increase their knowledge of anatomy. In physiology Albrecht van Haller, a student of Boerhaave's, investigated breathing and digestion. In the USA, in 1822, William Beaumont had a patient whose stomach was opened by gunshot. He was able to observe the digestive system at work. None of this, however, resulted in doctors discovering the real cause of disease.

There was also some important work in surgery, as well as the contribution of John Hunter (see box). William Cheselden (1688–1752) found a way of removing a stone from a bladder in just over a minute! Such speed was welcomed, given the lack of effective anaesthetics at this time.

HERMANN BOERHAAVE

Hermann Boerhaave was the Professor of Medicine at Leyden, in Holland, between 1718 and 1729. He taught his students to keep case histories and carry out post-mortems to try to establish causes of death. He taught the need to make use of science and the experience of the patient rather than just rely on abstract theory. His students moved on to other parts of Europe and to America, spreading his ideas. One of these, Alexander Monro, turned Edinburgh University into a leading medical centre.

JOHN HUNTER

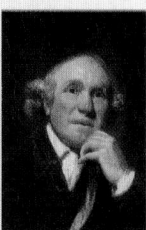

John Hunter (1728–93) has been called the 'Father of Modern Surgery'. His brother, William, was a famous surgeon. John went to London to work for him in his dissecting rooms. He trained as a doctor. He worked as a surgeon in St George's Hospital and, for a time, became an army surgeon. He built up a collection of anatomical specimens from people and animals which formed the basis of the Royal College of Surgeons' collection. John invented new procedures, like **tracheotomy** to clear air passages. He also investigated transplanting teeth.

10.1 THE OLD ORDER BEGINS TO CHANGE **75**

Source A

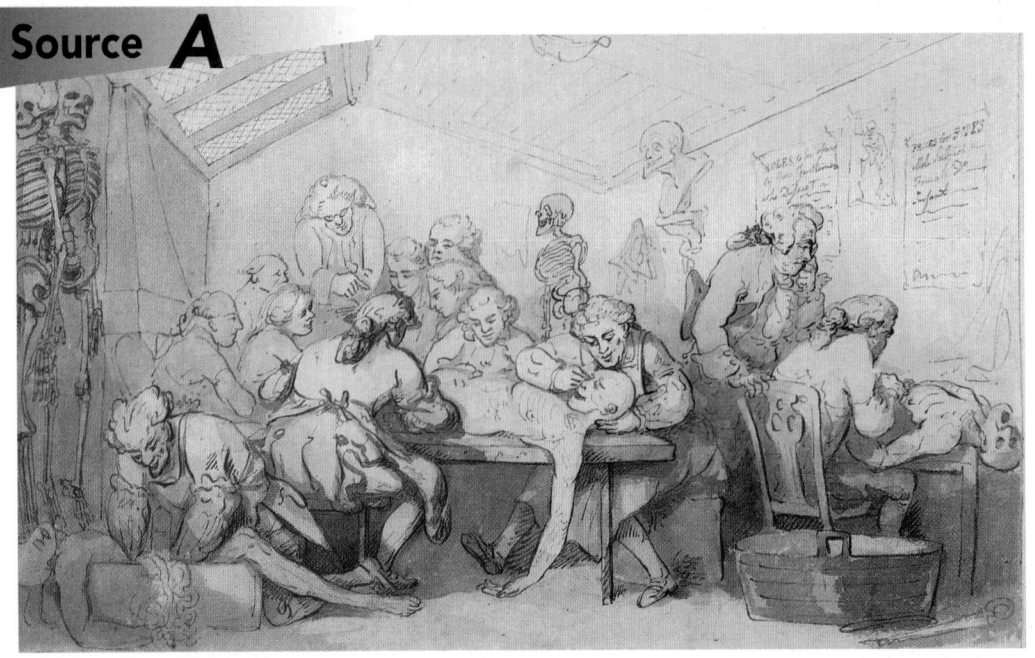

◄In the 18th century, surgeons based their work on an increasing knowledge of anatomy and pathology. This drawing, by Thomas Rowlandson, shows William Hunter's dissecting room in the latter half of the 18th century.

The medical profession became more respected during the 18th century. Surgeons at last gained equal status with physicians. Organizations were set up in Britain and Europe to represent surgeons. The Company of Surgeons was established in 1745 and, in 1800, it became the Royal College of Surgeons of London. This set the standards for surgical training. People were beginning to feel that society should care for its members. Several new hospitals were founded at this time by rich people, including Guy's in 1721 and the Middlesex Hospital in 1745.

'Quackery'

Despite the search for new knowledge, many old ideas continued in use during the 18th century. Many doctors still clung to the four humours and their associated treatments. To explain the mystery of how disease spread, many adopted the idea of 'miasmas' (colourless, odourless gases in the air which spread infection). 'Quack' doctors, in search of profit, peddled all sorts of nonsense. For example, 'piss-prophets' emphasized diagnosis by examining urine. Other 'quacks' recommended useless pills or claimed that evil worms caused illness. A German doctor, Franz Mesmer (1734–1815), claimed that he could cure patients by hypnotism.

Source B

►This picture of doctors was drawn by William Hogarth, an 18th century artist. They are sniffing the gold tops of their walking sticks which contain a liquid they thought would prevent infection. One doctor is tasting some patient's urine.

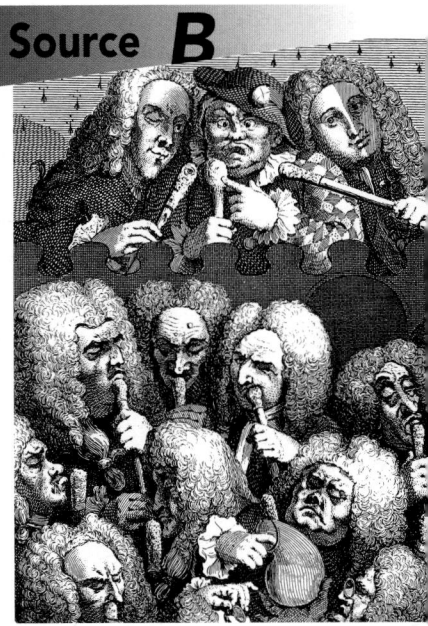

QUESTIONS

1 During the 18th century it was fashionable to question and inquire. What effect did this attitude have on medicine?

2 Despite this attitude why did many old ideas continue in use?

10.2 The situation in 1820

Despite the advances of the 17th and 18th centuries medical practice and knowledge was still limited.

- People still did not know what really caused disease. Doctors had an insufficient knowledge of chemistry and biochemistry. There was also a lack of technical aids for doctors. Although microscopes were in existence, they were not very powerful. Further developments in physics were needed if they were to be improved.

- Surgical operations were still carried out in filthy conditions as surgeons did not realize the need for cleanliness. Infection, therefore, was rife. Operations had to be carried out in haste because there were no effective anaesthetics. Patients often died from the trauma of the pain. Blood loss during an operation was another problem. Although surgeons knew there was a problem with losing too much blood, they were unable to carry out successful transfusions. They were not aware at this time that there were blood groups which had to be matched.

By the early 20th century, however, most of these problems had been overcome. How and why was this able to happen?

THE GROWTH OF INDUSTRY

First Phase: late 18th – 19th century
- **1781** James Watt perfected the steam engine. This enabled machinery to be powered effectively. The need for new machinery meant the growth of an engineering industry.

- **1840s** Rapid extension of the railway network. Travel and communications quicker.

- **1850–75** Britain was the 'workshop of the world'. It was later challenged by the USA, Germany and France.

Second Phase: late 19th century
New light industries were developed:
- the motor car
- giant chemical firms
- electrical engineering
- new materials came into use such as steel, rubber and aluminium.

Third Phase: 20th century
Society moved into the age of high-technology. New machines invented to aid medicine. For example:
- **1896** X-ray machines
- **1945** kidney dialysis machine
- **1970** body scanners.

10.3 The impact of the Industrial Revolution

In the late 18th century a number of changes took place which turned Britain into an industrialized society. The population began to increase rapidly and there was an increase in demand for all types of goods. Factories that were full of machines sprang up. These machines were powered at first by water, then by steam and latterly by electricity.

Around the factories large towns grew up very rapidly. Initially this brought slum housing, poor public health and epidemics of infectious diseases.

On the other hand, industrialization stimulated the rapid development of the sciences and technology. New machines and new materials were brought into use. For example, a deeper knowledge of physics and improvements in glass-making led to the manufacture of more powerful microscopes. This, in turn, was a vital factor in scientists discovering that germs caused disease. Once this breakthrough was made new cures and vaccines followed.

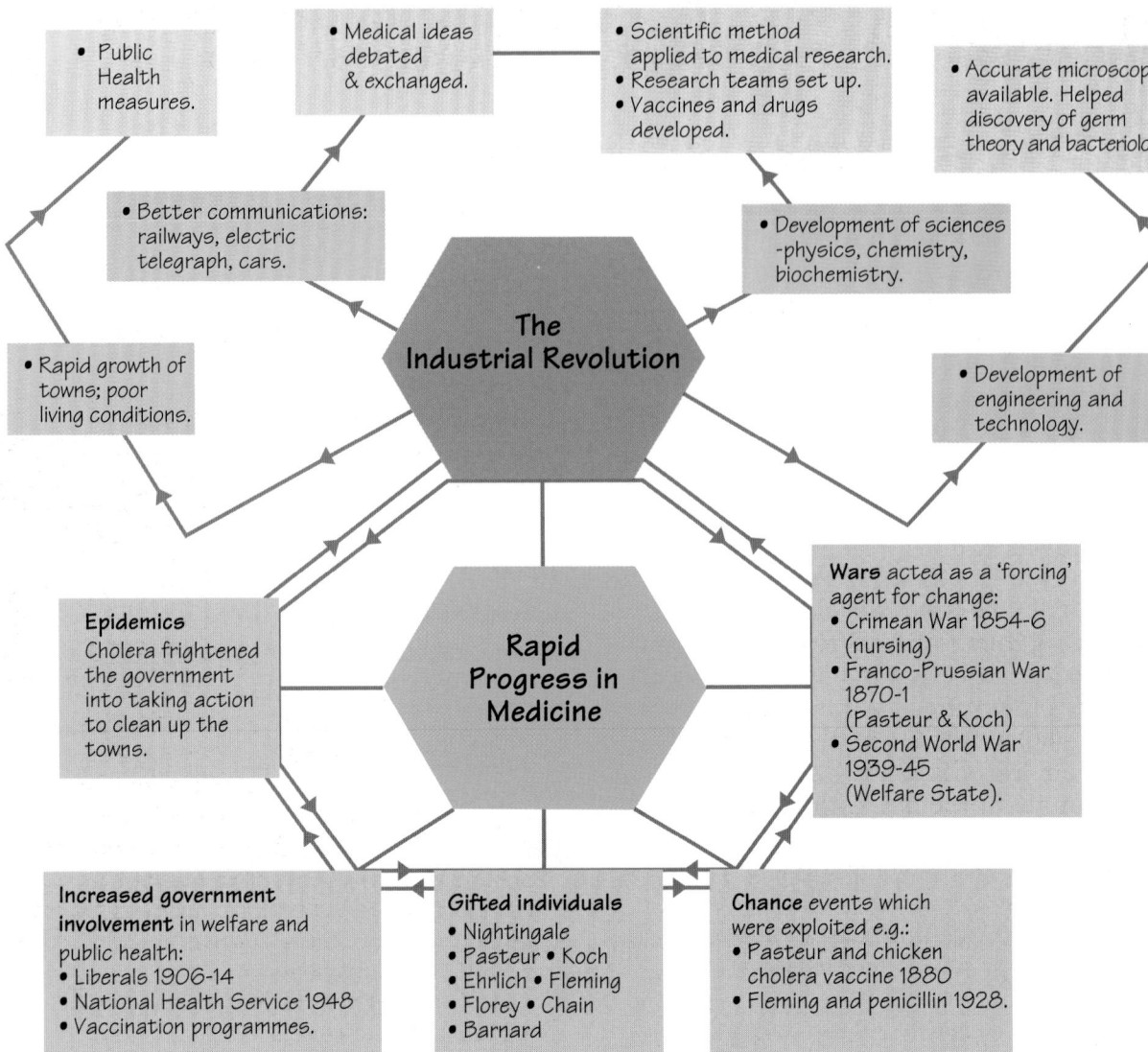

▲ **The web of factors which enabled medicine to progress very quickly after about 1850.**

The diagram contains:

- Public Health measures.
- Medical ideas debated & exchanged.
- Scientific method applied to medical research.
- Research teams set up.
- Vaccines and drugs developed.
- Accurate microscopes available. Helped discovery of germ theory and bacteriology.
- Better communications: railways, electric telegraph, cars.
- Development of sciences -physics, chemistry, biochemistry.
- Rapid growth of towns; poor living conditions.
- Development of engineering and technology.

The Industrial Revolution

Rapid Progress in Medicine

Epidemics Cholera frightened the government into taking action to clean up the towns.

Wars acted as a 'forcing' agent for change:
- Crimean War 1854-6 (nursing)
- Franco-Prussian War 1870-1 (Pasteur & Koch)
- Second World War 1939-45 (Welfare State).

Increased government involvement in welfare and public health:
- Liberals 1906-14
- National Health Service 1948
- Vaccination programmes.

Gifted individuals
- Nightingale
- Pasteur • Koch
- Ehrlich • Fleming
- Florey • Chain
- Barnard

Chance events which were exploited e.g.:
- Pasteur and chicken cholera vaccine 1880
- Fleming and penicillin 1928.

Chemistry also made advances during this period. Chemists, working in teams, began research into drugs.

When electricity came into use in the late 19th century it opened the way for new machines and technical aids to help medicine.

As well as industrialization other factors were also at work (see diagram). Combinations of these factors enabled medicine to progress very quickly from the mid-19th century, compared with the slow pace of change over the previous 3,000 years. This rapid progress – sometimes called the medical revolution – is dealt with in the next three chapters.

QUESTIONS

1 What problems faced medicine in 1820?

2 Why has there been such rapid progress in medicine since about 1850?

3 Which of the factors in the diagram had influenced medicine before 1820? Give examples and details.

THE FIGHT AGAINST INFECTIOUS DISEASE

11.1 Edward Jenner and smallpox

The first significant step in the fight against infectious disease was made in 1796, with the discovery of a vaccine to protect people from smallpox.

During the 18th century smallpox had taken over from the plague as the major killer disease. Victims suffered from a high fever and sores full of pus appeared all over the body. If the heart, brain and lungs became infected, death was certain. Some people who survived were left disfigured and, often, blinded. Many had tried to make themselves **immune** from smallpox by the risky practice of inoculation. This involved deliberately infecting themselves with the disease, taken from someone who was suffering from a mild form of it. By doing this they hoped that they would catch a mild form of smallpox too.

Edward Jenner (1749–1823) was a doctor from Berkeley in Gloucestershire. He studied under John Hunter, the famous surgeon, and from him learned the importance of scientific observation and experiment. Hunter once advised Jenner, 'don't think, try the experiment'. Jenner was aware of the local belief that milkmaids who suffered from the mild disease of cowpox, never caught the dreaded smallpox. Years of observation confirmed this belief. So, in 1796, he decided to move on from observation to experiment. For the experiment to work he had to use a person who had never had cowpox or smallpox. He chose a young boy, James Phipps, and injected him with pus from the sores of Sarah Nelmes, a milkmaid with cowpox. Phipps developd cowpox. When he was fully recovered, Jenner gave him a dose of smallpox. If the experiment worked all would be well. If not, Phipps would develop smallpox and probably die.

The experiment worked (see Source A). Jenner had found a way to make people immune from a deadly, infectious disease without the risks of inoculation. He called his method vaccination, after the Latin word *vacca* which means 'cow'.

INOCULATION

Lady Mary Wortley Montagu learned of inoculation against smallpox when she was in Turkey with her husband, the British ambassador. In 1718 she introduced the idea into England. A cut

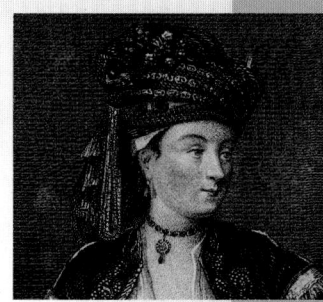

was made in the patient's arm and a thread soaked in pus from the sores of a victim who had a mild form of the disease was drawn through. The patient was kept in a warm room until the symptoms had disappeared. Inoculation became popular but some patients died as they contracted a fatal form of the disease. Inoculation houses were set up and some doctors, like William Woodville, became famous and wealthy from the technique.

Source A

I selected a healthy boy, [James Phipps] about eight-years old. The cowpox matter was inserted into the arm of the boy on 14 May 1796. On the seventh day he complained of uneasiness, on the ninth day he became a little chilly, lost his appetite and had a slight headache but next day he was perfectly well. Then he was inoculated with smallpox, but no disease followed.

▲ **Edward Jenner, writing about his vaccination experiment in 1798.**

The reaction to Jenner's discovery

Despite the success of Jenner's experiments, some doctors were against vaccination. This was because they either did not want to accept new ideas or they had a vested interest in supporting inoculation. They had become rich and famous from this technique and feared that they would lose everything to the new methods of an unknown country doctor. Jenner, however, had powerful supporters. Some members of the royal family were vaccinated. Vaccination was widely accepted abroad. A group of Native Americans travelled to Britain to thank Jenner. In 1813 the Emperor Napoleon released a prisoner of war at Jenner's request. 'Ah, it's Jenner, I can refuse Jenner nothing!' the Emperor said. In 1802 Parliament gave Jenner £10,000 and in 1806 a further £20,000. In 1840 vaccination was made free for all infants and, in 1853, it was made compulsory. This was especially surprising at a time when the government usually refused to interfere in people's lives, even for the good of their health. Smallpox was on the way to being defeated, even though nobody had the faintest idea how vaccination worked. It was to be 80 years before another vaccine was discovered.

Source B

27 October 1793 – John Moore Paget was inoculated with smallpox.

26 January 1834 – Baby Margaret was vaccinated by Mr Drake, the smallpox being at Mells and Downhead.

25 June 1844 – Jane did not go out on account of Richard who was not so well, but leeches and warm baths relieved him.

▲ Extracts from the unpublished diaries of the Paget family of Cranmore, Somerset.

▼ This cartoon, drawn by James Gillray in 1802, shows the supposed fears of some people at the time about Jenner's use of cowpox matter as a vaccine against smallpox.

Source C

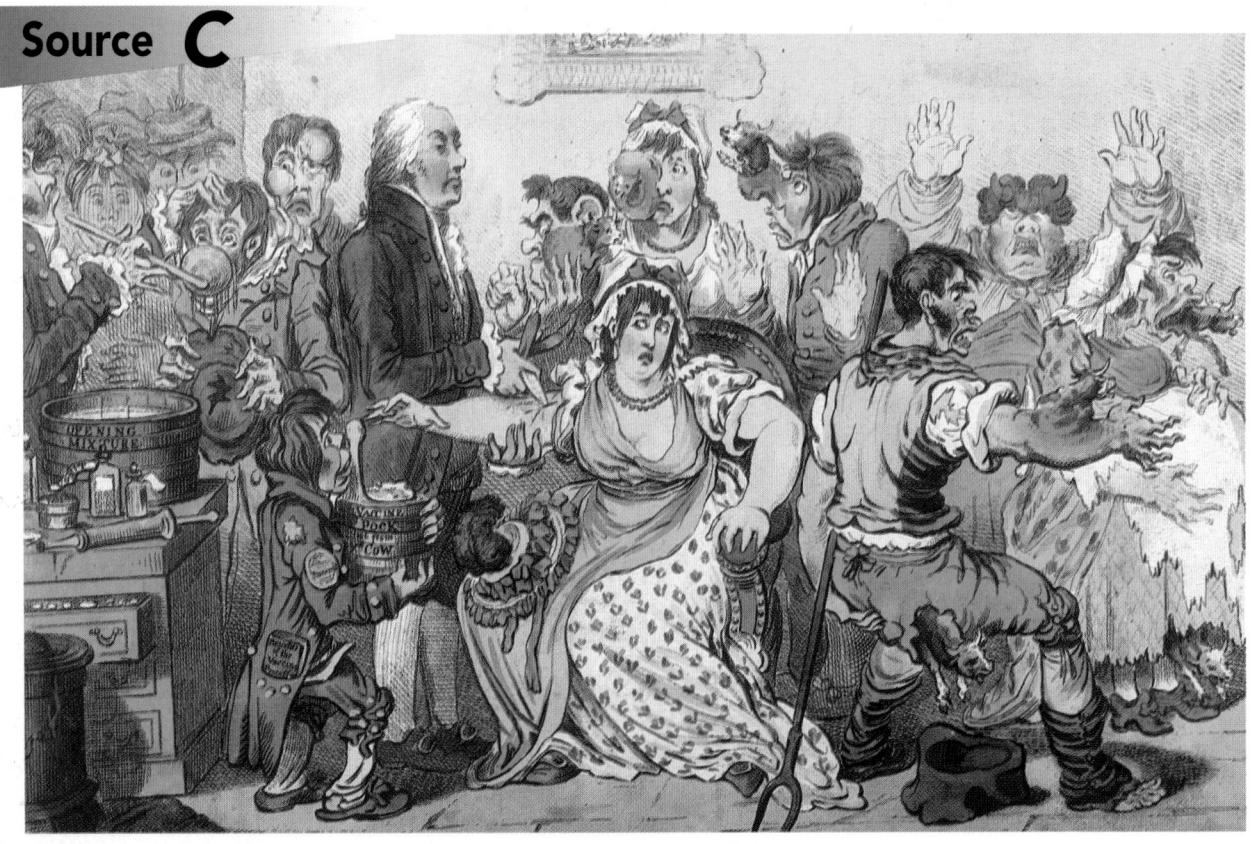

Source D

In August 1799 John Ring from Wincanton in Somerset met Dr Jenner. In 1808 he went to Ringwood, Hampshire, to investigate supposed failures of vaccination. Feelings ran so high that his group had to carry pistols for defence. When the British Vaccine Establishment was opened in 1809, Ring was the principal vaccinator. He vaccinated so many that Jenner, speaking of a lady who had vaccinated ten thousand people, said that it was nothing compared to honest John Ring.

▲ From *The History of Wincanton* by George Sweetman, 1903.

Source E

After being vaccinated with cowpox she was so ill with fever, and with these boils, that she could not work for a week. Many years later she caught smallpox.

▲ An account by C. Cooke, an apothecary from Gloucester, of a patient whose vaccination failed to give protection from smallpox, 1799.

Source F

This day is published, price one shilling [5p], a letter from John Birch, Esquire. In this publication it is noticed that there was a Parliamentary grant of £30,000 to Dr Jenner for an unsuccessful experiment. There is also a letter proving the production of a new and fatal disease called the 'vaccine ulcer' described by Astley Cooper, Esquire, surgeon of Guy's Hospital. There is a letter from Mr Westcott of Ringwood proving the failures of the experiment there. A list of those who died of cow pox there. A list of those who were defectively [ineffectively] vaccinated and caught smallpox; and those who died of smallpox after having been vaccinated and told that they would be protected. There is also a list of other failures under the Treatment of the Jennerian Institution.

▲ Opposition to Jenner and the smallpox vaccination shown in a contemporary letter.

Source G

Medicine has never before produced any single improvement of such usefulness. You have erased from the list of human afflictions one of the greatest. Future generations will only know through history that the loathsome smallpox has existed and has been wiped out by you.

▲ A letter to Edward Jenner from Thomas Jefferson, President of the USA, 1802.

SUMMARY

► Smallpox was a feared epidemic disease in the 18th century.

► Inoculation was introduced into Britain by Lady Mary Wortley Montagu. Though popular, it was risky and did not reduce the toll from smallpox.

► Jenner saw that cowpox victims became immune from smallpox.

► He vaccinated people with cowpox which made them immune to the disease.

► Opposition was overcome because vaccination worked, was widely publicized and had many supporters.

► Jenner had no idea how or why vaccination worked, so his work did not lead directly to other developments.

QUESTIONS

1 Study Source B. How does it show
   a change and
   b continuity in medical practice?

2 What factors led to Jenner's success with the smallpox vaccine?

3 a Describe what is shown in Source C.
   b Would a historian find this source useful?

4 a Why was there opposition to vaccination?
   b How was this opposition overcome?

5 Was Jenner's discovery a **change** or a **development** in the history of medicine? Explain your answer.

Progress in the fight against infectious diseases by 1900

By 1900 the germs which caused the most common diseases had been discovered. Koch, Pasteur and others had developed a number of vaccines that could prevent people from catching these diseases. Governments were also introducing preventative measures against disease by enforcing councils to provide clean water and efficient sewage disposal. Doctors and scientists now needed to find effective cures for people with infectious disease.

There was some knowledge to build on. Drugs made from natural substances had been used for centuries in the treatment of illness. For example, opium was used as a pain-killer and colocynth as a purgative. These drugs, however, were unable to combat the bacteria which caused the disease. By about 1890, the work of Joseph Lister was accepted by most doctors. Lister showed that a chemical, carbolic acid, would kill germs outside the body – but it was too toxic to use internally. A chemical that could be used safely to kill bacteria inside a person was needed. In 1900 the conditions were ripe for a breakthrough in curative medicine to be made – but who was going to make it?

Paul Ehrlich

By the late-19th century, the German chemical industry was progressing rapidly, particularly in the manufacture of synthetic dyes. Koch was experienced in using synthetic textile dyes to stain microbes for examination under the microscope. This made the microbes stand out and easier to study.

Paul Ehrlich was a German doctor who joined Koch's research team in 1889. He began by working with Emil Behring on diptheria and became fascinated by the fact that the body produced **antibodies** to ward off specific germs inside a person without damaging the rest of the body. He referred to such antibodies as magic bullets because, like a bullet from a gun, they sought out their specific target. Antibodies, however, did not always kill off invasive bacteria. Ehrlich began to think that there must be a chemical dye that could be used internally to kill specific bacteria without harming the rest of the body – a synthetic magic bullet.

The search for a magic bullet

Ehrlich became director of his own research institute. His team concentrated on looking for chemical cures for disease. In 1899 Ehrlich, and his team of researchers, started to test different dyes to see if they would kill microbes. This involved a great deal of patience and perseverance. Numerous dyes were tried but they met with only limited success. Dyes were found that attacked malaria and sleeping sickness germs.

PAUL EHRLICH

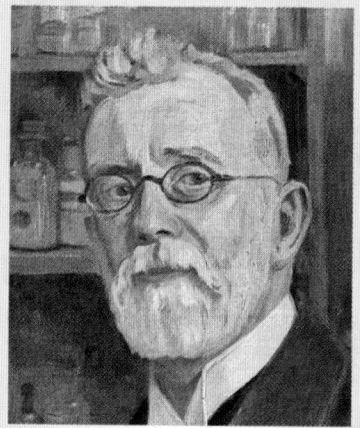

Ehrlich was born in the town of Strehlen in Silesia, Germany, in 1854. He studied at the University of Leipzig, researching in chemistry and bacteriology. He worked first as a doctor but, in 1886, caught tuberculosis (TB). It took him three years to recover completely. In 1889, he joined Robert Koch's research team at the Institute for Infectious Diseases in Berlin. He helped Emil Behring to find an anti-toxin that cured diphtheria. From 1899, until his death in 1915, he was the Director of the Royal Institute of Experimental Therapy in Frankfurt. It was here that he carried out his research into chemotherapy (the treatment of disease by chemical drugs). In 1908 he shared the Nobel Prize for medicine with the Russian bacteriologist Elie Metchnikov.

Salvarsan 606

◀ **Factors involved in the discovery of Salvarsan 606.**

The syphilis microbe

In 1906 the microbe that caused syphilis was identified by Fritz Schaudinn and Paul Erich Hoffman. Syphilis was a sexually transmitted disease which killed thousands of people each year. In 1907 Ehrlich decided to test chemical compounds of various poisons, hoping that one might kill the syphilis germ. His team made up and tested over 600 **arsenic** compounds. All of them were said to be useless. The research seemed to be going down a blind alley.

In 1909 Sahachiro Hata, a Japanese bacteriologist, joined Ehrlich's team. Hata was asked to retest the compounds already discarded. He found that compound 606 did in fact kill the syphilis germ. Why had it previously been ruled out? Perhaps the assistant who had previously tested the compound lacked concentration or was not such a skilled researcher. Ehrlich called the new drug Salvarsan 606. He was concerned that doctors might give the wrong dose, or that the drug might be harmful in other ways. He insisted on repeated testing on many hundreds of animals that were deliberately infected with syphilis. He found that it always targeted the syphilis germ without harming the rest of the body. Salvarsan 606 was used for the first time on a human patient in 1911.

Opposition

The discovery of Salvarsan 606 was not welcomed by everyone. Some doctors were not keen to use the new drug; it was not very soluble and was difficult and painful to inject into veins. Some doctors believed that people would become promiscuous now that they knew that syphilis could be cured. Despite Ehrlich's rigorous testing there were many doctors who did not like the idea of giving their patients arsenic, in any form.

QUESTIONS

1 a What progress had been made in the fight against infectious diseases by 1900?

 b What new breakthrough was needed?

2 a What factors enabled the discovery of Salvarsan 606 to be made?

 b Was any one of these factors more important than the others? Explain your answer.

3 a What opposition was there to Salvarsan 606?

 b Does your study of the history of medicine make you surprised that there was opposition to such an important breakthrough in the treatment of disease? Give reasons and examples in your answer.

Gerhard Domagk and sulphonamide drugs

Domagk worked for a large chemical firm in Elberfeld, Germany. Inspired by Ehrlich's work, he carried out a programme of systematic research looking for dyes that might destroy infecting microbes within the body. Domagk, like Ehrlich, was conscientious and determined.

His first success was the discovery of germanin, a drug which was effective against sleeping sickness. Then, in 1932, he discovered that a red dye, called prontosil, stopped the streptococcus microbe (which causes blood-poisoning) from multiplying in mice without harming the rest of the animal. He had no idea, however, whether this drug would work on humans. One day, in 1935, Domagk's daughter, Hildegarde, pricked herself with an infected needle and blood-poisoning set in. The girl was seriously ill and Domagk, with nothing to lose, gave her a huge dose of prontosil. Although her skin turned slightly red she made a rapid recovery.

Further research by a team of French scientists found that the compound in the dye which acted on the germs was sulphonamide, a chemical derived from coal tar. It was not long before other sulphonamide-derived drugs were developed that were capable of fighting diseases such as tonsillitis, puerperal fever and scarlet fever. In 1938, chemists working for the British firm, May and Baker, discovered a sulphonamide-derived drug that worked against the microbe causing pneumonia. They tried the drug on a Norfolk farm labourer, who had severe pneumonia, and it worked. They called the drug M&B 693, as it was the 693rd compound they tested before they met with success.

Sulphonamide drugs, however, had disadvantages. They sometimes caused damage to the kidneys and liver and were ineffective against the more virulent microbes. An even more powerful magic bullet was needed if infectious disease was to be conquered.

The story of penicillin

Penicillin was the world's first **antibiotic** – that is the first drug derived from living organisms, such as fungi, which would kill or prevent bacteria from growing. Penicillin was effective against a variety of germs. Its development involved three brilliant individuals: Alexander Fleming, Howard Florey and Ernst Chain.

Stage 1 1928

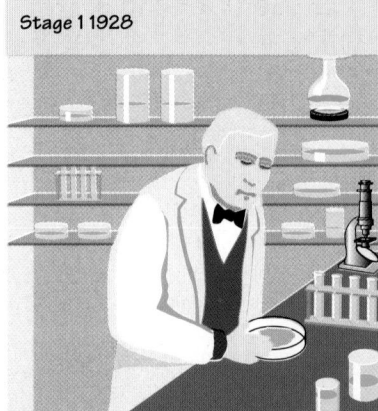

Alexander Fleming discovered the penicillin mould. He was unable to produce pure penicillin from the mould. He published a report of his work but did no more.

Stage 2 1938–41

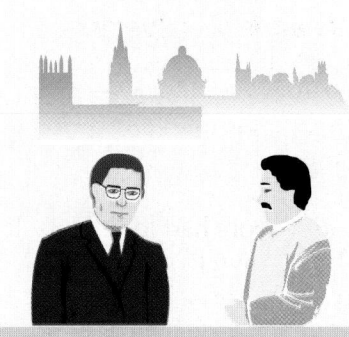

A team of researchers at Oxford University, led by Howard Florey and Ernst Chain, developed a method of making pure penicillin. They could not make large amounts however.

Stage 3 1941–44

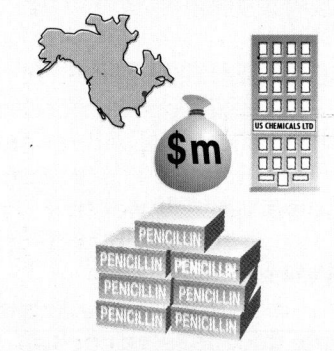

In 1941 the USA entered the Second World War. The US government funded research into methods of making large quantities of penicillin. By 1944 enough penicillin was available for Allied soldiers.

► **Stages in the penicillin story.**

Alexander Fleming's early life

Fleming was born in Lochfield, Ayrshire, in 1881. In 1902 he went to London to study medicine and, in 1906, was taken on as a research assistant in the Inoculation department at St Mary's Hospital, London. The department was led by Sir Almroth Wright, an eminent doctor who had discovered a vaccine against typhoid in 1896. Wright was now anxious to find new vaccines. During the First World War, Fleming worked in a military hospital in Boulogne, treating wounded soldiers. He was appalled to see that antiseptics such as carbolic acid did not prevent infection in deep wounds. After the war, Fleming returned to St Mary's determined to find a substance that could kill germs more effectively. In 1922 he discovered that a natural substance in tears, lysozyme, would kill some germs, but not those that caused disease and infection.

A chance discovery?

In 1928 Fleming was carrying out research into staphylococci (the germs which turn wounds septic). This involved growing the germs on **agar** in culture dishes. When Fleming came to clean a pile of discarded culture dishes, he noticed a mould spore had lodged itself on to one of them. It had grown to a size of about one centimetre across the dish. This was not an unusual thing to happen but Fleming was quick to notice that, around the mould, the germs had stopped growing. Another less astute person might have thrown away the dish and thought nothing more about it, but Fleming was curious. The mould was a member of the *penicilium notatum* family. It produced a bacteria killing juice which Fleming called penicillin.

He grew further quantities of the mould and found that it stopped other deadly germs growing, including anthrax and diphtheria bacilli. He injected it into animals without it harming them. However, if penicillin was to be of any practical use in treating humans, a way had to be found of turning the mould juice into a pure drug. Fleming and his colleagues were unable to do this. No one was prepared to give them the specialist help or money to carry out further experiments. Fleming wrote up his findings and published articles in the *British Journal of Experimental Pathology* in 1929 and 1931. He did nothing more about his discovery.

Source O

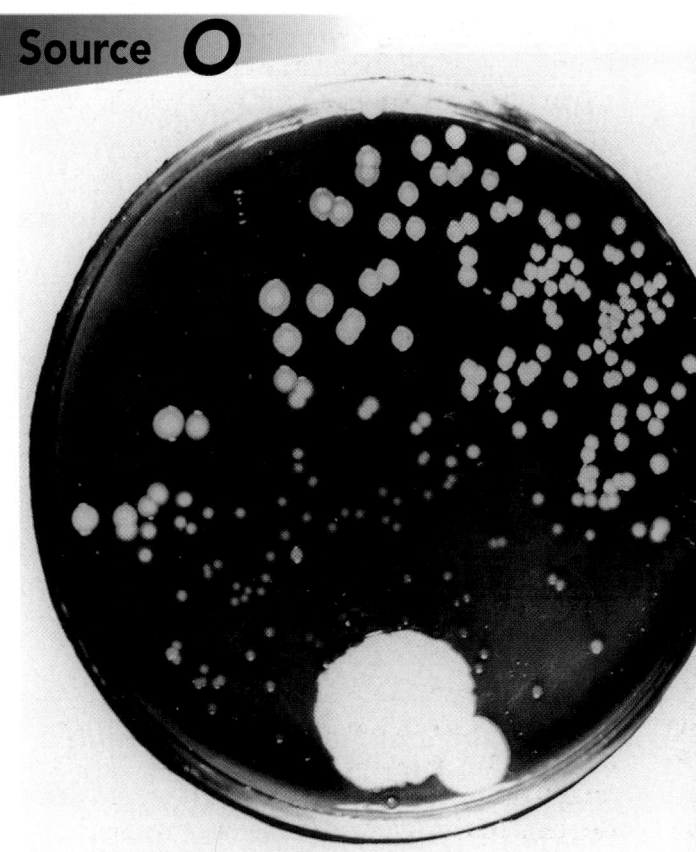

▲ The dish with the 'abnormal' culture that caught Fleming's attention. The mould can be seen on the left. On the right, germs can be seen growing in large numbers, but near the mould there is a clear area.

Howard Florey and Ernst Chain

In 1935 Howard Florey, an Australian doctor, became the head of the William Dunn School of Pathology at Oxford. He built up a team of brilliant biochemists to carry out medical research, including Ernst Chain, a scientist who was a refugee from Germany. Chain, who was Jewish, came to Britain to escape from Nazi persecution. In 1938 Florey's team decided to study germ-killing substances. Chain came across Fleming's articles on penicillin and they decided to see if they could produce pure penicillin from the mould juice. They succeeded in making small quantities of pure penicillin in powder form and decided to test it out on animals. On 25 May 1940 eight mice were injected with streptococci. Four were then given regular doses of penicillin and they survived. The other four mice all died within sixteen hours. Florey claimed that they had witnessed a miracle.

Problems in the production of pure penicillin

Florey's team did not have the resources to manufacture the pure penicillin in large amounts. They grew the mould in milk bottles, bed pans and milk churns and turned it into pure penicillin using a a process of freeze-drying devised by Chain. In October 1940 they tried it out for the first time on a human – a policeman, Albert Alexander, who was suffering from blood-poisoning and close to death. He began to recover after receiving penicillin, only to die when supplies ran out.

War and the US chemical industry

The curative qualities of the drug were now beyond question. But mass producing the drug for commercial use still remained a problem. Only large chemical companies, with their resources could solve the problem, but it was unlikely they would be willing to get involved. By this time, Britain was deeply engaged in the Second World War against the might of Nazi Germany. The British chemical industry was too busy producing explosives to become involved in the manufacture of penicillin.

Florey realized that penicillin would be able to cure the deep infections caused by war wounds. He decided to visit the USA to try and persuade American chemical firms to invest in the mass production of penicillin. To begin with, he was unsuccessful. Then, in December 1941, the USA entered the war after the Japanese attacked Pearl Harbour. Soon, the US government had made grants available to firms wishing to buy expensive equipment to make penicillin. Mass production by British firms began in 1943. By 1944 sufficient penicillin was available to supply all the needs of the Allied forces. After the war more efficient processes for the mass production of penicillin were invented. The cost of the drug was reduced and it became used across the world to treat a whole range of diseases.

The Fleming 'myth'

In August 1942 a friend of Alexander Fleming's lay dying in St Mary's Hospital. Fleming contacted Florey in Oxford and asked for some penicillin to treat his friend. Florey immediately obliged and the patient made a rapid recovery. The story appeared in *The Times* and, on 30 August 1942, Almroth Wright wrote a letter to the newspaper saying that Fleming was the person responsible for the drug. People began to believe that the development of penicillin was due entirely to Fleming. Even though Florey and Chain were awarded the Nobel Prize, along with Fleming in 1945, their part in this incredible medical breakthrough was played down.

Source P

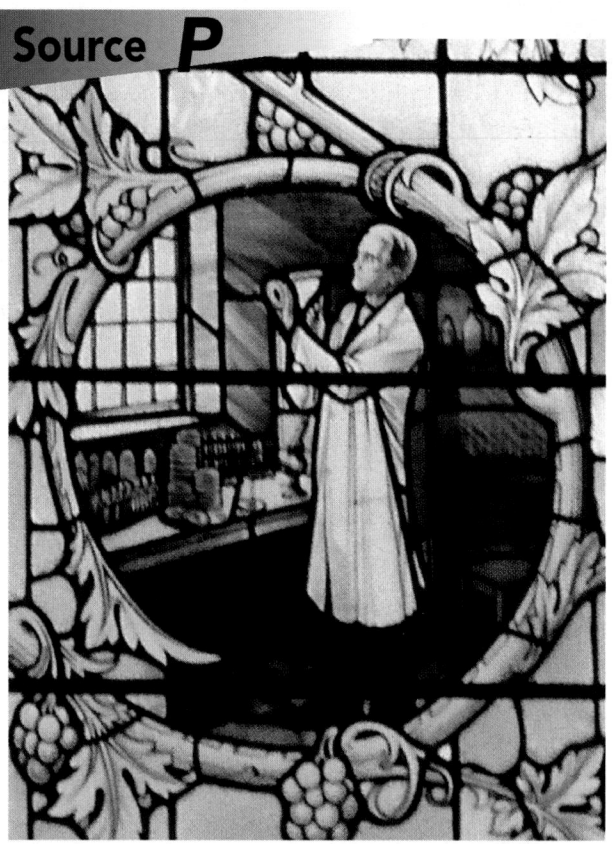

▲ This stained glass window, showing Alexander Fleming at work in his laboratory, was installed in St James' Church, Paddington, London. The church is very close to St Mary's Hospital, where Fleming had worked for 49 years.

Source **Q**

Sir In your article on penicillin yesterday you refrained from putting the laurel wreath for this discovery around anyone's brow. I would supplement your article by pointing out that it should be decreed to Professor Alexander Fleming of this laboratory. For he is the discoverer of penicillin and also the author of the original suggestion that this substance might ...have important applications in medicine.

▲ Extract from the letter written to *The Times* by Sir Almroth Wright. It was published on 30 August 1942.

Source **R**

There has been a lot of most undesirable publicity in the newspapers and press about penicillin. The whole subject is presented as having been foreseen and worked out by Fleming. This steady propaganda seems to have its effect even on scientific people, in that several have now said to us, 'But I thought you had done something on penicillin too'.

▲ Extract from a letter written by Howard Florey to Sir Henry Dale in December 1942. Dale was the President of the Royal Society, a body concerned with the advancement of science and medicine.

QUESTIONS

1 Louis Pasteur once said that 'chance favours the prepared mind'. Was the discovery of penicillin in 1928 a matter of good fortune?

2 What part did the following factors play in the penicillin story:

  a the brilliance of individual scientists
  b teamwork
  c war?

3 a What is the Fleming 'myth'?
  b How did it come into existence?
  c Who do you think deserves the credit for penicillin: Fleming or Florey and Chain? Give reasons for your answer.

4 Would penicillin have been discovered even if Fleming, Florey and Chain had not lived? Explain your answer.

Has infectious disease been conquered?

Penicillin and similar antibiotics have been hugely successful in fighting infection. Today the main killer diseases, especially in the developed industrialized countries, are non-infectious; cancer and heart disease being the most serious. However, infectious disease has not been fully conquered. Some bacteria have become immune to antibiotics such as penicillin. Scientists and governments are still searching for a vaccine and cure for **AIDS**. Tuberculosis, contrary to popular belief, has not been wiped out. In 1990 it was responsible for the deaths of 1.8 million people, mainly in the developing world.

There are also other problems do with ethics. Large companies make huge profits out of selling drugs. Some drugs, such as **thalidomide**, went on to the market, without being fully tested so that all the side effects could be identified. Following this, in 1964, the British Government established the Committee on Safety of Drugs to screen all newly developed drugs.

SUMMARY

► **1891** Behring discovered that anti-toxin serum could be used to cure diphtheria in humans.

► **1909** Ehrlich and Hata discovered a new chemical drug, Salvarsan 606, which kills the syphilis germ. This was the first chemical 'magic bullet'.

► **1932** Domagk discovered prontosil – the second magic bullet and first of the sulphonamide drugs.

► **1928** Fleming discovered penicillin – the first antibiotic. He did not go on to develop it further.

► **1938** Florey and Chain began their research into the production of pure penicillin at Oxford.

► **1942** The US chemicals industry invested in the mass production of penicillin, so that it was readily available to the Allied forces in the Second World War.

Source 1

Pasteur was a small man capable of inspiring devotion in others. He also had aggressive manners which could make people who were equally as clever both bitter and enemies. One of his strongest motivations was to show how much more clever he was by destroying their arguments entirely. **Nationalism** was a powerful force in his life. He wanted to work for the glory of France. He worshipped the French Emperor, Napoleon III. When France and Prussia [part of Germany] went to war in 1870, his hatred of the Germans was intense. Personal ambition was very important to him. He wanted to be famous.

▲ **This opinion of Pasteur was written by Robert Reid in *Microbes and Men*, 1974.**

Source 2

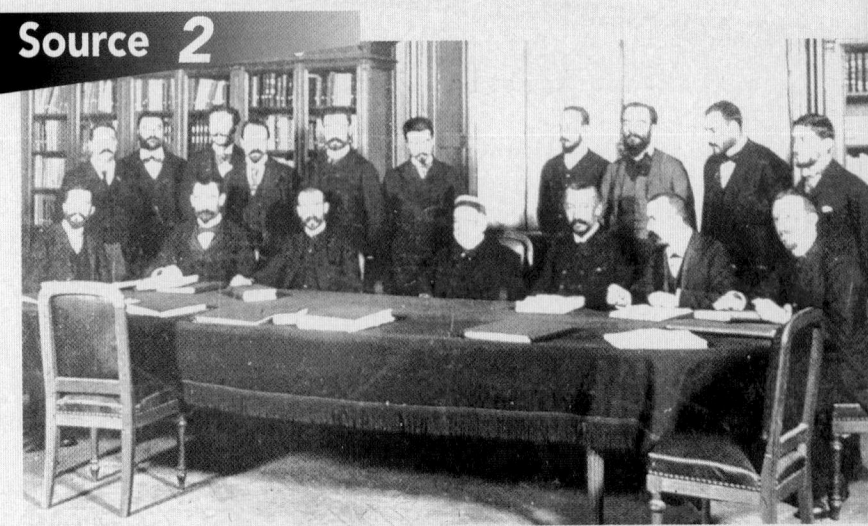

▲ **Pasteur and his team. Dr Emile Roux, his main assistant, is seated on his right. Albert Calmette who, together with Camille Guerin, discovered a vaccine against TB in 1906, is seated on the far right of Pasteur.**

Source 3

At the International Conference of Hygiene in Geneva, 1882, Koch left Pasteur in no doubt that he believed that Pasteur had contributed nothing new to science. Pasteur lost his temper and years of hatred came out. Yet Pasteur's work had been the great idea. Koch's scientific skill had made its application possible.

▲ **Robert Reid's analysis of the conflict between Pasteur and Koch in *Microbes and Men*, 1974.**

Source 4

I am very satisfied with the success of the experiments with the rabid dogs. You must keep a careful check on the dogs and a daily written record of what happens to them, making absolutely certain whether they become ill or not, or if they should be cured.

▲ **From a letter written to Eugene Viala by Louis Pasteur, 6 September 1883. Viala was a member of Pasteur's team and was assisting in the research on the rabies vaccine.**

1 a Study Sources 1, 2 and 4. What factors can you find that enabled Pasteur to make his discoveries?
  b What other factors contributed to Pasteur's achievements?

2 Was the proof of the germ theory a turning point in the development of medicine? Explain your answer.

3 'Louis Pasteur was the most important individual in the fight against infectious disease'. Do you agree or disagree with this statement? Explain your answer.

CHAPTER 12

THE REVOLUTION IN SURGERY

12.1 Anaesthetics conquer pain

Problem of pain

Surgeons had long had to face the problems of pain, infection and bleeding. This was still true in the early 19th century. There were no effective anaesthetics. Surgeons gave their patients drugs like opium and mandrake, or tried to get them drunk. A few surgeons used 'mesmerism' (hypnosis), hoping the patient would ignore the pain. Surgery had to be quick. Deep internal operations were out of the question. Most surgery was limited to removing growths or amputating limbs. Even so, many patients died from the trauma of the excruciating pain.

During the late 18th century the science of chemistry had made some progress. In 1772 Joseph Priestley, an English chemist, discovered that oxygen was a gas. Other chemists were also investigating the properties of different substances. In 1799 Humphrey Davy (1778–1829) discovered pain could be relieved by inhaling nitrous oxide ('laughing gas'). He wrote a pamphlet saying that nitrous oxide might be successfully used as an anaesthetic by surgeons. The medical profession, however, ignored his suggestion.

Anaesthetics are drugs given to a patient to make surgery pain free.
There are two types:

General anaesthetics – these are drugs which are usually inhaled and render the patient unconscious.

Local anaesthetics – these are usually injected and have the effect of numbing one particular part of the body such as a tooth. They do not make the patient unconscious.

Source B

A patient preparing for an operation was like a condemned criminal preparing for an execution.

▲ From a letter written to James Simpson in 1848, by a man who had undergone surgery before effective anaesthetics.

Source A

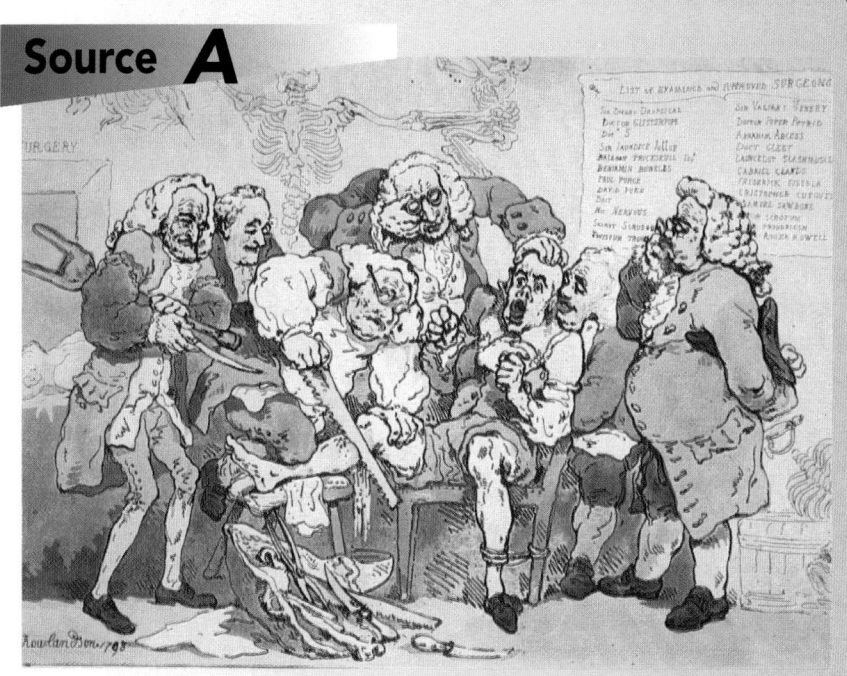

LIST OF EXAMINED AND APPROVED SURGEONS

◄ A cartoon drawn by Thomas Rowlandson, showing an operation in 1793. The list of doctors' names on the wall shows that the cartoonist saw doctors as more concerned with money than with caring for their patients.

Early successes

During the early 1840s a number of experiments were made to find an effective anaesthetic. In 1842 the American doctor, Crawford Long, found that ether was a useful anaesthetic, but did not publicly announce his discovery.

On 10 December 1845 an American dentist, Horace Wells, saw people inhaling nitrous oxide at a fair. He noticed that they could injure themselves, but felt no pain. The next day, Wells had a tooth painlessly taken out after inhaling the gas. He tried to demonstrate painless tooth extraction to some medical students at a Hospital in Boston, USA. What he did not know was that some people are not affected by nitrous oxide. Wells' volunteer yelled as the tooth was taken out. The students left shouting 'Humbug! Humbug!'

On 16 October 1846 William Thomas Green Morton (1819–68) persuaded John Warren, the head surgeon at the Boston Hospital, to carry out an operation in public using ether as an anaesthetic. The patient, Gilbert Abbott, was given ether through an inhaler by Morton. Warren proceeded to remove a tumour painlessly from his neck. Warren turned to his audience and announced: 'Gentlemen, this is no humbug!'

News of Warren's success spread quickly to Europe. By 18 October, a Dr Bigelow, who had seen the operation, had published an article on it. On 3 December a steamship carried a letter from Bigelow to a Dr Boot in London. By 19 December Dr Boot had extracted a tooth using ether – and had written an article about it. On 21 December the surgeon, Robert Liston, successfully amputated the leg of Frederick Churchill (a butler) using ether as an anaesthetic. Liston removed the leg in 26 seconds! With the leg already on the floor, Churchill raised his head and asked Liston when he was going to begin the operation.

Source C

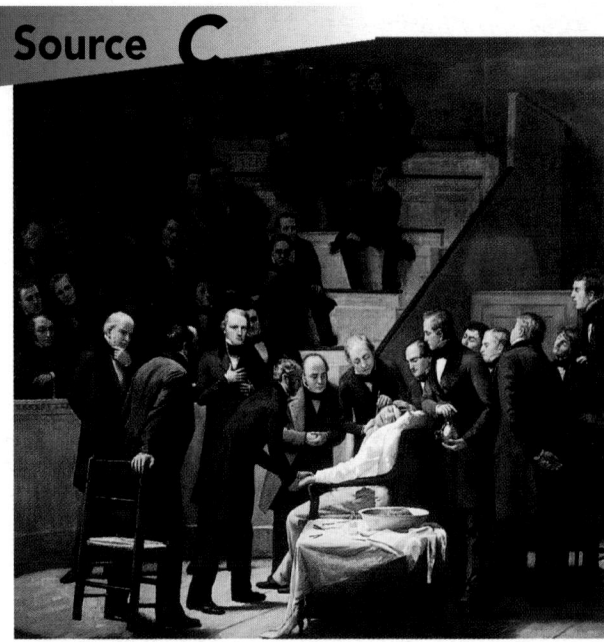

▲ Warren's operation on Gilbert Abbott, 16 October 1846, painted by Robert Hinckley in 1882.

Source D

This Yankee dodge, gentlemen, beats mesmerism hollow!

▲ A remark made by Robert Liston to the audience after his public operation on Frederick Churchill at the University College Hospital, London.

QUESTIONS

1 What problems of surgery are shown in Source A?

2 Make out a chart, like the one below, to record the times when experiments were made with anaesthetics.

Date	Event	Person(s) involved

3 Source C is a painting completed after the event. Is it a reliable source of evidence for a historian? Explain your answer.

4 Study Source D. What do you think Liston meant?

James Simpson and chloroform

James Young Simpson (1811–70), Professor of Midwifery at Edinburgh University, wanted to find something which relieved pain during childbirth. He disliked ether because it was inflammable, had a pungent smell and, when inhaled, irritated the lungs making the patient cough. He began to test the effects of different chemicals. On 4 November 1847 Simpson and two other doctors discovered the effects of chloroform (see Source E). Simpson found chloroform easier to administer than ether. Less of it was needed and it appeared to take effect more quickly. By the end of November he had given chloroform to more than 50 patients and he declared himself pleased with the outcome.

Opposition to anaesthetics

These anaesthetics meant painless operations, but they were not welcomed by everyone.

- Some people worried that surgeons were too inexperienced. They were unsure as to the correct amount to give or of any side effects they could have. There were even instances of explosions in operating theatres caused by the use of ether. Their fears appeared to be realized when, in 1848, Hannah Green, aged fifteen, died from an overdose of chloroform. Deaths also occurred from the overuse of ether.
- Members of the Calvinist Church in Scotland were outraged at the use of chloroform in childbirth. They pointed to the Book of Genesis where God says to Eve: 'In sorrow shalt thou bring forth children.' In other words, God intended women to bear pain when giving birth.
- Some people were worried that anaesthetics placed the patient under the total control of the surgeons. What if they did something against the patient's will?
- In the army some officers regarded the use of anaesthetics as 'soft'. In 1854 John Hall, Chief of Medical Staff in the Crimea, told his team of doctors: 'A good hand on the knife is stimulating. It is much better to hear a fellow shouting with all his might than to see him sink quietly into his grave.'

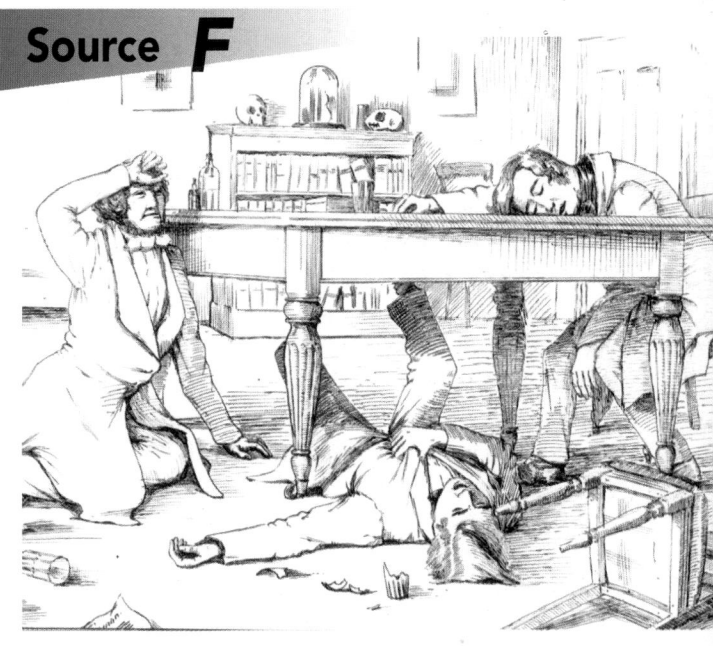

The royal seal of approval!

Some of this opposition disappeared when, on 7 April 1853, Queen Victoria was given chloroform during the birth of her eighth child, Prince Leopold. The anaesthetist was Dr John Snow, later to do vital research into cholera. The Queen wrote in her journal that chloroform was 'soothing, quietening and delightful beyond measure.' Chloroform became socially more acceptable as a result of the Queen's experience. It became the most popular anaesthetic until about 1900, when it was realized that it could damage the liver. Surgeons then returned to using ether.

Anaesthetics from the late 19th century to the present day

Even though anaesthetics came to be accepted, there were still problems in using them. Massive amounts were often needed, not to prevent pain, but to relax the muscles. Patients became saturated and slept for hours, even days. Recovery was slow and there were frequent complications.

From the end of the 19th century, anaesthetists became specialists. New substances were discovered and put into use. In 1884 cocaine was first used as a local anaesthetic, numbing one part of the body while the patient remained conscious. In Germany, in 1905, novocaine was proved to be more effective than cocaine. In 1942 curare, a South American poison, was first used as a muscle relaxant during operations; it remains in use today. A skilled anaesthetist is now a crucial member of the surgical team, responsible for monitoring the patient's well-being during operations.

Source G

▲ A chloroform inhaler from 1879. It consists of a cotton facemask on to which the chloroform was poured.

QUESTIONS

1 Why did Simpson dislike ether?

2 Does Source E show that chance played a part in the discovery of chloroform?

3 What other factors enabled Simpson to make his discovery?

4 a Why was there such fierce opposition to anaesthetics?

   b How was this opposition overcome?

Source H

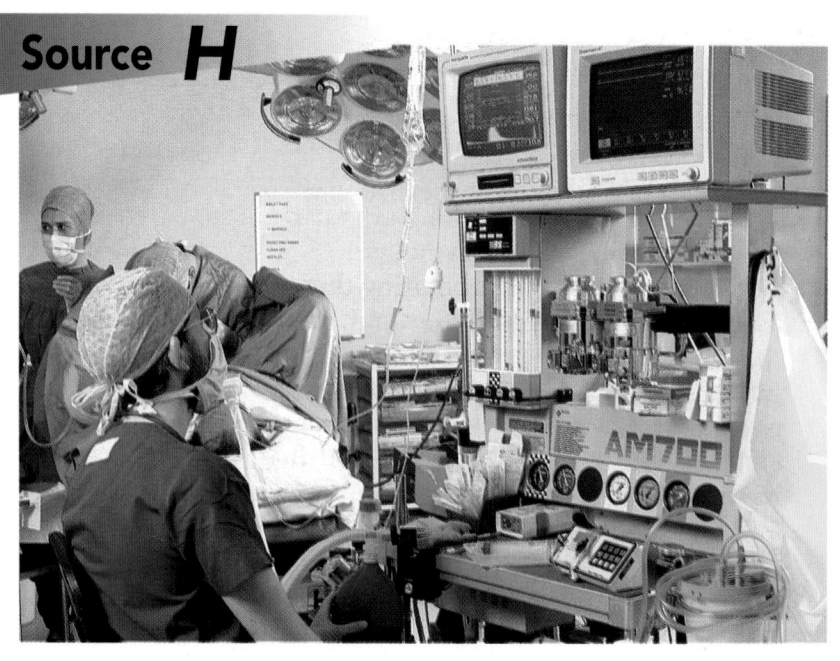

▶ Modern anaesthetists at work. Anaesthetists now monitor heart beat, blood pressure, breathing patterns and brain waves using high-technology equipment.

The problem of infection

The period between the first use of ether as an anaesthetic in 1846 and about 1870 has been called the 'black period' of surgery. The removal of pain made surgeons over confident and they performed many operations that they would not have attempted before anaesthetics. Operations, however, were still carried out in unhygienic conditions. Surgeons wore their everyday clothes when operating and instruments were not sterilized between operations. Before Pasteur proved the germ theory the need for cleanliness was not understood. As a result, many patients died from the infections that developed after the operation.

Ignaz Semmelweiss

Semmelweiss was a young Hungarian doctor working in Vienna in the 1840s. He was worried about the high death rate of women from puerperal fever, an infection which set in after childbirth. Some doctors believed this was spread by miasmas present in the air of hospital wards. In 1847 Semmelweiss suggested that the doctors themselves might be spreading the infection by examining patients immediately after dissecting the dead bodies of victims of the disease. He ordered the doctors to wash their hands in a solution of chloride of lime before examining patients. This was unpleasant and many doctors resented it. But the death rate from puerperal fever in these wards fell dramatically. Other doctors did not accept Semmelweiss' method. The high death rates continued in most places.

Joseph Lister and antiseptics

The breakthrough in preventing infection was made by Joseph Lister. He had read of Pasteur's research and he realized that the infections that were killing his patients were caused by germs. To kill any germs that were present he decided to use carbolic acid, a disinfectant that was used to combat the smell at sewage works. He knew that the smell of rotting sewage and the operating theatre were similar. First he used bandages soaked in the acid, then he developed his technique to include a spray that drenched the air, the surgeon's hands, the instruments and the patient. This was unpleasant for surgeons but the results were remarkable. Mortality plummeted and when Lister died in 1912, ten times as many operations were being performed as there had been in 1867. Surgeons were able, for the first time, to operate without fear of infection killing the patient. The combination of anaesthetics and antiseptics meant that surgery was now much safer.

JOSEPH LISTER
(1828–1912)

Joseph Lister came from a well off family in Essex. By the time he was 33, he was Professor of Surgery at Glasgow. Although, at first, many doctors opposed his ideas, Lister was recognized for making one of the greatest advances ever in surgery.

The figures below come from his records of amputations.

Date	No. of patients	% died
1864–6 (no antiseptics)	35	46%
1867–70 (antiseptics)	40	15%

Source 1

Lister's creativity was a simple process. Chance had not helped in his discovery. He had read of the germ theory of disease and had applied it. The only significant piece of luck involved was the sweeping effects of the consequences. Millions of lives were saved by the new principle of **antisepsis** [the use of antiseptics to kill germs] and what followed it. The frightful spectre which had haunted operating theatres had at last been shown to have an organic cause, and Lister had shown how to defeat it.

▲ Robert Reid, *Microbes and Men*, 1974.

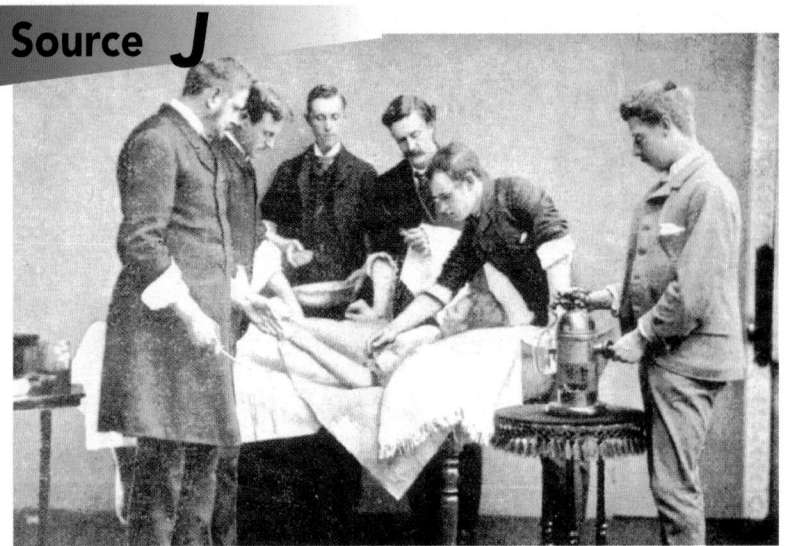

An antiseptic operation in Aberdeen in the 1880s. Lister's steam carbolic spray is being used.

Despite the [support] of statistical evidence, Lister's method met with interference and even violent opposition . . . Fully twenty years of patient trial, improvement, demonstration and education were needed before British surgeons were won over to the idea, and not before many senior members of the profession had been replaced by a younger generation.

Leo M. Zimmermann and Ilza Veith, *Great Ideas in the History of Surgery*, 1961.

From antiseptic to aseptic surgery

Antiseptic surgery had its drawbacks, not least being the discomfort felt by surgeons and nurses whose skin was burnt by the carbolic acid and lungs irritated by the spray. Rather than trying to fight germs, surgeons in Germany developed techniques for keeping them away. This is known as **asepsis** and aseptic surgery quickly became the normal procedure in the operating theatre. The idea of scrupulous cleanliness originated with Professor Neuber and was developed by Ernst Bergmann. Surgeons' hands, clothes and instruments were all sterilized. A chamber was used to pass superheated steam over the instruments, thus killing the germs without the need for disinfecting chemicals.

The 'father' of American surgery, William S. Halsted, introduced a further innovation. In 1889 his nurse, Caroline Hampton, complained that antiseptic chemicals were harming her hands. Halsted asked the Goodyear Rubber Company to make some gloves. He had a particular interest as he was to marry Nurse Hampton in 1890. Halsted realized that the gloves were protecting the patient as well as the nurse. He followed this by introducing caps, masks and gowns for surgery. Halsted also investigated cocaine as

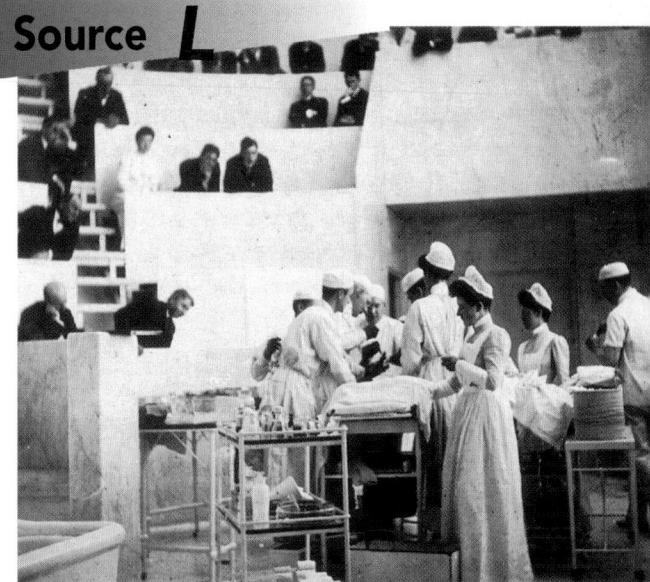

Halsted in the operating theatre at the Johns Hopkins Medical School, Baltimore, USA. He operated and taught his students at the same time.

an anaesthetic but became a drug addict, taking both cocaine and morphine.

Today instruments are pre-packed in sterile containers. The air is sterilized before it enters the operating theatre. Some operations, especially on babies or for joint replacement, take place in sterile 'tents' to ensure that there is no risk of infection.

The problem of bleeding

The idea of replacing lost blood had been considered for several centuries. A French mathematician and doctor, Jean-Baptiste Denys, transfused blood from a lamb to a mad young man in 1667. The man lived but the next patient died and the practice was prohibited. In 1818 doctors in London successfully transferred blood from human to human. Most transfusions were disastrous as the red blood cells in the patient's blood clumped together and the patient would die from this reaction to the donor's blood.

Yet the need to replace lost blood became more and more important as surgery expanded due to anaesthetics and antiseptics. Patients were still dying from massive blood loss. This problem was overcome in 1900, when Karl Landsteiner discovered that blood was divided into groups. Some of these could not be mixed with other groups as clumping would occur. Once blood groups were understood, successful transfusions were possible. Clotting on contact with air was solved when the use of sodium citrate was discovered during the First World War (1914–18). Blood could then be taken and kept for later use. In 1938 the National Blood Transfusion Service was set up in Britain. During the Second World War, donors often saw it as their patriotic duty to stock blood banks.

Plastic surgery

Grafting skin to repair damaged features was practised in ancient India and during the Renaissance but infection was a major problem. The development of new weapons in the 20th century meant that the number and type of facial and skin wounds increased. In Britain, Harold Gillies set up a unit to treat horrific wounds inflicted during the First World War. He was the first plastic surgeon to consider the patient's appearance. Gillies' assistant was a New Zealander, Archibald McIndoe. In the Second World War, McIndoe set up a unit at East Grinstead in Sussex where he treated over 4,000 patients, mostly airmen, whose faces and hands were disfigured by blazing petrol. His patients, known as 'guinea pigs', were helped by developments in drugs like sulphonamides and penicillin that helped prevent infection. Plastic surgery has become a vital branch of surgery, bringing better quality of life to people whose lives would otherwise be shattered by injury or birth defects.

Source M

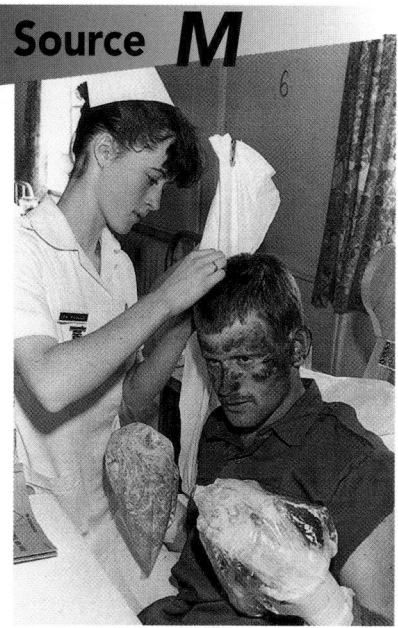

▲ A serviceman with extensive burns receives the latest plastic surgery skin graft techniques, Falklands War, 1982.

Source N

One hundred and fifty years ago, patients would only lie on the operating table in desperation when they were tortured by agony from their gangrenous leg or stones in the bladder. Now with modern anaesthesia, with antiseptics, with blood transfusion, with antibiotics - the modern miracles of surgery - nothing can escape. Everything, from the brain to bunions, is available for the surgeon's healing knife.

▲ A comment made by Professor Harold Ellis of Westminster Hospital to a group of medical students in the BBC television programme, *The Courage to Fail*, in 1987.

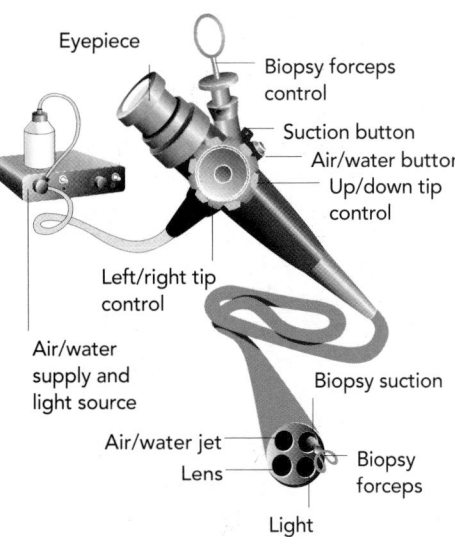

Eyepiece

Biopsy forceps control

Suction button

Air/water button

Up/down tip control

Left/right tip control

Air/water supply and light source

Biopsy suction

Air/water jet

Lens

Light

Biopsy forceps

▲ Endoscopes using fibre optics are used to examine and diagnose virtually every hollow tube in the body.

Source O

During the mid-1960s, I remember wards having forty beds. They were called Nightingale Wards. They had a family feeling because patients after an operation spent seven to ten days there and got to know each other. On the days when surgery was performed I often stood in front of a patient who was having the operation to shield the performance from onlookers on a double decker bus outside who strained to see what was happening. The surgeon and anaesthetist would often parade around the ward to see that all was well. No one changed out of their surgical gowns so bloodstained chaps in white wellington boots would be seen coming up the ward on most days. During visiting time we packed up and sterilized all the instruments for the next day's operations. We even cleaned the wheels on the beds.

▲ Denise Simpson remembers her first years as a nurse in Somerset.

High technology surgery

Surgeons could often benefit from the rapid development of science and technology in the late 19th and 20th centuries. The increasing use of electricity meant that many machines could be developed to assist surgery. Plastics and steel enabled artificial joints to be made for replacement surgery.

In 1895 Wilhelm Röntgen, professor of physics at the University of Würzburg, discovered X-rays. These enabled surgeons to look at the inside of a patient without making any incision. Marie and Pierre Curie discovered a new element, radium, in 1898. This eventually led to improved treatment for cancer. In 1903 the first electrocardiograph was developed by Willem Einthoven. Eventually it enabled surgeons to monitor the heartbeat effectively. The first artificial kidney machine was developed in 1943 by the Dutch surgeon, Willem Kolff. The first successful operation with a heart-lung machine, which enabled the heart to be stopped long enough for an operation to be carried out, took place in 1953.

Efficient microscopes for surgeons to use when operating were developed in the 1960s. Along with fine **sutures** and needles, they made it possible for doctors to join microscopic nerves and blood vessels and even to reattach severed limbs. One strange result of the development of microsurgery was the reintroduction of leeches in the 1980s because they are efficient in keeping blood flowing in an affected limb.

The development of **fibre optics** has enabled surgeons to examine the inside of the body and to operate without the risks of invasive surgery and major incisions. They can now reach the upper part of the body through the mouth or the bowels, via the rectum, without cutting the patient open. 'Keyhole' surgery allows patients to suffer less trauma, to have a local rather than a general anaesthetic and to recover more quickly.

▼ A surgeon using an endoscope to look inside the patient. It is inserted through a small incision near the patient's navel.

Source P

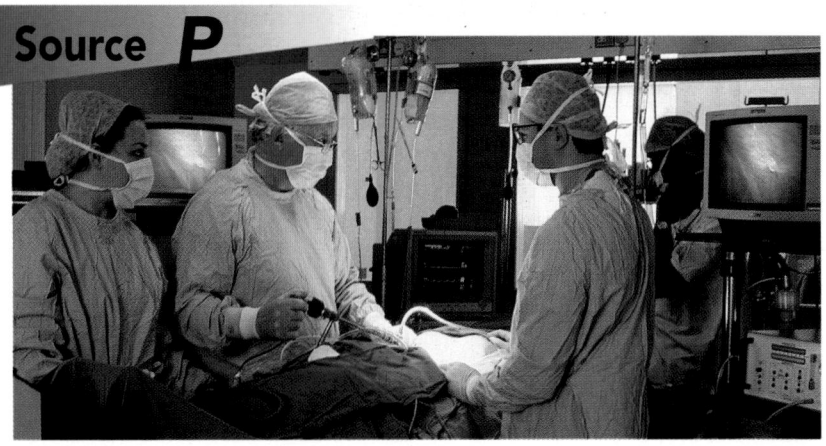

Heart surgery

Before the Second World War, surgery on the heart was dangerous and rarely carried out. When surgeons opened the chest, the patient's lungs collapsed and when the heart was touched, it stopped. It was thought that nothing could be done about this.

The Second World War provided the stimulus to further research as some soldiers had bullets and fragments of shrapnel lodged in their hearts. A US army surgeon, Dwight Harken, had the courage to try to save them. He cut into the beating heart and stuck in his finger to remove the fragments. This made little difference to most patients who needed open heart surgery to correct defects. The problem was that the blood supply needed to be cut off when the heart was opened. After four minutes, this caused brain damage. A Canadian surgeon, Bill Biggelow, came up with the idea of lowering the patient's body temperature to gain more time. Nevertheless the problem remained.

At the University of Minnesota, Norman Shumway led a team specializing in pioneering heart surgery but there was sometimes a 50 per cent death rate. In 1960 the Methodist Hospital in Houston, Texas, became the centre for heart surgery under Michael de Blakey. He worked at immense speed and used knitted Dacron, an artificial fibre, to replace diseased arteries. The problem of transplanting a replacement heart remained. Tissue rejection made it seem impossible. However, research continued despite the shortage of human hearts. In 1967 Norman Shumway announced that he was ready to try a human heart transplant. In New York, Dr Adrian Kantrowitz prepared to operate on a baby on 3 December. That same morning he heard that Christiaan Barnard had performed the world's first human heart transplant.

Source Q

Of the first group of fourteen operations, all the patients died. In the second group of fourteen, seven died and in the third group two died. In the fourth group all the patients lived. The difference was that the first three groups were experimental animals, the fourth group were injured soldiers.

▲ A description of Dwight Harken's operations on injured hearts.

Source R

Administrators decided we were spending too much. They had the enormous stupidity to suggest that, if we kept patients out, we could work within budget. I said, 'No problem. We've got a shot gun. I'll load it. You fire it, because that's what you're planning. Now, out.'

▲ Denis Melrose, a leading British heart surgeon, describing a difficulty he faced in the 1960s.

Source S

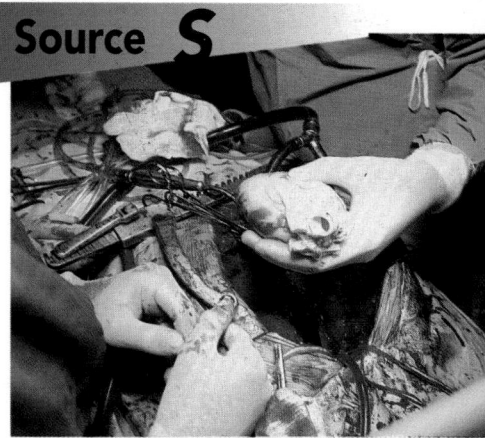

▲ The heart is an organ that was difficult to operate on. Advances in technology meant heart-lung machines could allow surgeons to work on the heart.

CHRISTIAAN BARNARD

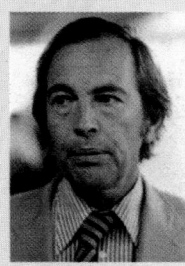

Christiaan Barnard was a surgeon at the Groote Schuur Hospital, Cape Town, South Africa, who studied heart surgery at the University of Minnesota. After returning to South Africa he set up a cardiac unit in Cape Town. In 1967 he transplanted the heart of a female road accident victim into 59 year old Louis Washkansky. There was press hysteria and Barnard became a public celebrity. However, Washkansky died after eighteen days from pneumonia as the drugs used to prevent his body rejecting the heart wiped out his resistance to infection.

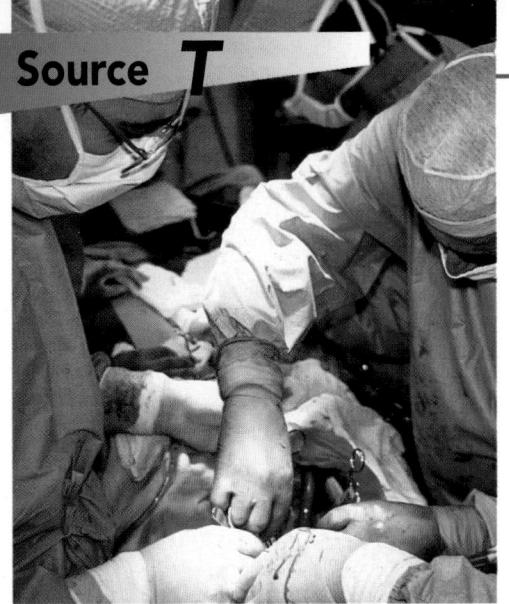

▲ An open heart operation. While the surgeons work on the opened heart of the patient, a heart-lung machine takes over the circulation of the patient's blood and provides oxygen for the blood. Before the invention of this machine, surgeons could not operate on the heart for more than a few minutes.

SUMMARY

▶ The combination of anaesthetics and antiseptics, developed by Joseph Lister, meant that surgery became much safer after 1870.

▶ Aseptic surgery, when no germs are ever allowed to be present, soon replaced antiseptic surgery.

▶ The discovery of the different blood groups allowed safe transfusions thus reducing the risks from blood loss in surgery.

▶ Surgeons began to specialize as surgery became safer. Plastic, brain and heart surgery were developed by pioneering individuals.

▶ Developments in science and technology contributed to new techniques in medicine.

▶ The wars fought in the 20th century speeded up developments in surgery.

Christiaan Barnard

Surgeons in the USA were disappointed, as they felt that they had done all the experimental work and Barnard had used their ideas. He denied this. Shumway and Kantrowitz carried out their operations but their patients soon died. Barnard did another transplant and his patient lived over a year-and-a-half. In Texas, Michael de Blakey and Denton Cooley also tried human transplants. Cooley was able to complete a transplant operation in twenty minutes. No one, however, could overcome the problems caused by the patient's immune system. The drugs the patients needed to get the body to accept the donor heart, left them open to infection. They always died within a relatively short time.

Enormous public expectation had been shattered. The failure rate was too high. Barnard tried to keep transplants going but did not succeed. Some saw him as the villain. Heart transplant operations ceased. Some doctors turned to experimenting with artificial hearts and, in 1982, Barney Clarke was given a plastic heart in Salt Lake City, USA. He died three weeks later.

The solution arrived by chance. In 1974 a researcher in Norway looking for new drug substances in soil samples came across the drug cyclosporin. It was found it controlled tissue rejection but did not eliminate all resistance to disease. Cyclosporin had a more dramatic effect on heart transplant surgery than the skills of Barnard and Cooley combined because it meant that transplants were possible again. By 1987, 90 per cent of patients lived more than two years. Heart transplants are now routine. Surgery, drugs, patient care and the control of rejection all interlink to give success.

QUESTIONS

1 Study Source I (page 66), Source J (page 100) and and Source T (page 104). What changes in surgery do they show?

2 Study Source O on page 102. In what ways had surgery changed since the 1860s?

3 **a** How important have individuals been in the development of surgery since 1870?
b How has science and technology helped surgery develop since 1870?
c What other factors have played a part in the development of surgery since 1870?

4 Some books claim that Christiaan Barnard made the most important breakthrough in the history of heart surgery. On the evidence in this chapter, do you agree?

In 1850, nursing was looked upon as a lowly occupation. Nurses were generally portrayed as uneducated and slovenly and they had a reputation for heavy drinking. This image, however, was not totally fair. The conditions under which they worked were often appalling and there was no proper training available. At Kaiserwerth in Germany, however, the local pastor, Theodor Fliedner, set up a small hospital and training school in 1853. He insisted that his nurses be of 'good character'. Elizabeth Fry, famous for her attempts to reform prison conditions in London's Newgate gaol, visited Kaiserwerth in 1840. She was so impressed that on her return to England she founded Britain's first nursing school, the Institute of Nursing Sisters. During the second half of the 19th century nursing underwent a revolution and developed into a respected profession. How did this change come about?

The Crimean War (1854–6): a tale of two women

Florence Nightingale (1820–1910) came from a wealthy middle-class family. In 1844 she told her parents that she wanted to enter nursing. Her parents naturally had a low opinion of nurses and it took Florence seven years of determined effort to persuade them to agree. She then visited Kaiserwerth, travelling on to Paris to study nursing. In 1853 she became the Superintendent at the Institution for the Care of Sick Gentlewomen in Harley Street, London which she ran very efficiently. By now she was fully committed to a career involving the training of nurses.

In March 1854 Britain, along with France and Turkey, went to war against Russia. The war was fought in the Crimea, a peninsula on the Black Sea, three thousand miles from Britain. A scandal broke when the public read the reports of William Russell, the war correspondent of *The Times* newspaper. He told of chaotic conditions in the Barrack Hospital in Scutari near Constantinople. Wounded British troops were being kept in overcrowded and filthy conditions. There were no nursing staff, no bandages and men were dying in agony.

Nightingale's work at Scutari

The Secretary of War, Sidney Herbert, who was a friend of the Nightingale family, wrote to ask Florence if she would 'go and superintend the whole thing'. She agreed to Herbert's request and, in the autumn of 1854, departed for Scutari in Turkey with a team of 38 nurses whom she had personally selected. When they arrived in Scutari, they were not warmly welcomed by the army doctors who felt that female nurses were 'unfavourable to military discipline and to the recovery of the patients'. Despite this undercurrent of hostility, Nightingale made sure that the wards were clean, the patients well fed, the sanitation and water supply improved and that supplies were plentiful. By early 1856 the death rate in the hospital had fallen from 42 per cent to 2 per cent.

Source U

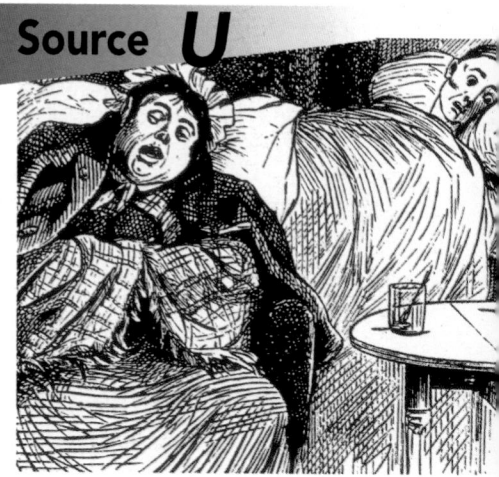

▲ This illustration shows how nurses were often portrayed in the 19th century – old and unattractive and possibly drunk.

Source V

She was a woman of iron will and imposed her ideas of nursing and medical care on those in authority and on her nurses. She had friends in the high place of the Cabinet. Through an endless stream of letters... she determined to improve nursing education and care... It can only be said that she succeeded mightily, in that every nurse, every patient, every hospital design, the organization of medical and nursing services everywhere, owe something to her... spirit.

▲ Philip Rhodes, *An Outline History of Medicine*, 1985.

Source W

She was a wonderful woman …All the men …would seek her advice and use her herbal medicines, in preference to reporting themselves to their own doctors …Her never failing presence among the wounded after a battle and assisting them made her loved by the rank and file of the whole army.

▲ Memories of Mary Seacole by a British soldier who fought in the Crimean War.

The work of Mary Seacole

Mary Jane Seacole (1805–81) was born in Kingston, Jamaica. Her mother ran a boarding house for invalid soldiers where Mary helped to care for the patients. In 1854 she went to England and told the War Office she was willing to go to the Crimea as a nurse. She was rejected and felt that it was because her 'blood flowed beneath a somewhat duskier skin than theirs'. In other words she was a victim of Victorian racism.

Not to be outdone, she made her own way to the Crimea and at her own expense. She set up a medical store and hostel near Balaclava, where soldiers could obtain medicines. She also tended the wounded on the battlefield and became known to the troops as 'Mother Seacole'. She met Florence Nightingale on several occasions but was not invited to join her team of nurses.

Seacole's fortunes after the Crimean War

In 1856 Mary Seacole returned to England but not to a heroine's welcome. She went bankrupt and received a deal of sympathy from the English press, notably *The Times* and *Punch* magazine. A four day festival of music was organized for her benefit in 1857, but it raised only £233. In the same year, Mary published her lifestory (see Source Y) in an effort to raise money. Although she was quite well-off when she died, no one in the medical world had bothered to make use of her nursing skills since the end of the Crimean War.

Source X

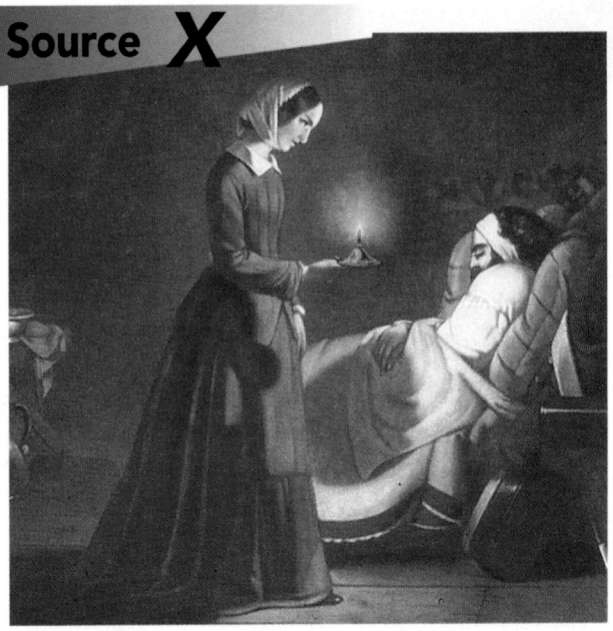

▲ A legend grew up around Florence Nightingale. She became known as 'the lady with the lamp' and 'an angel of mercy'. She was said to tour the wards at night making sure the patients were comfortable. This picture was painted by Tomkins in 1855.

Source Y

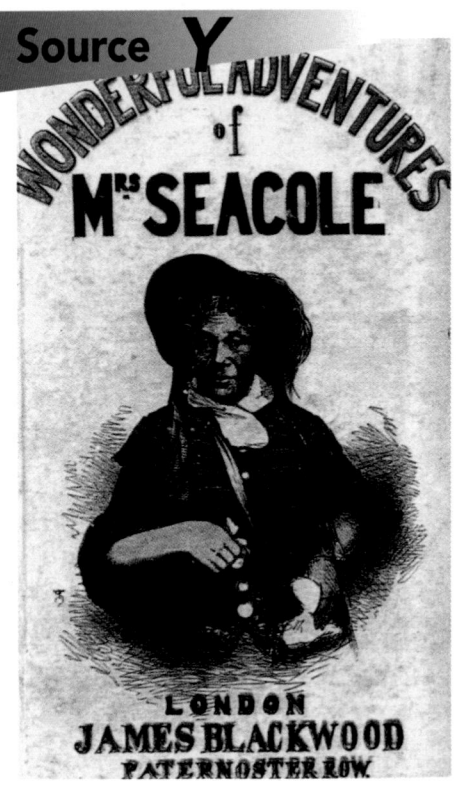

WONDERFUL ADVENTURES of Mrs SEACOLE

LONDON
JAMES BLACKWOOD
PATERNOSTER ROW

▲ A rare portrait of Mary Seacole. It appears on the title page of her autobiography, *The Wonderful Adventures of Mrs Seacole*, published in 1857.

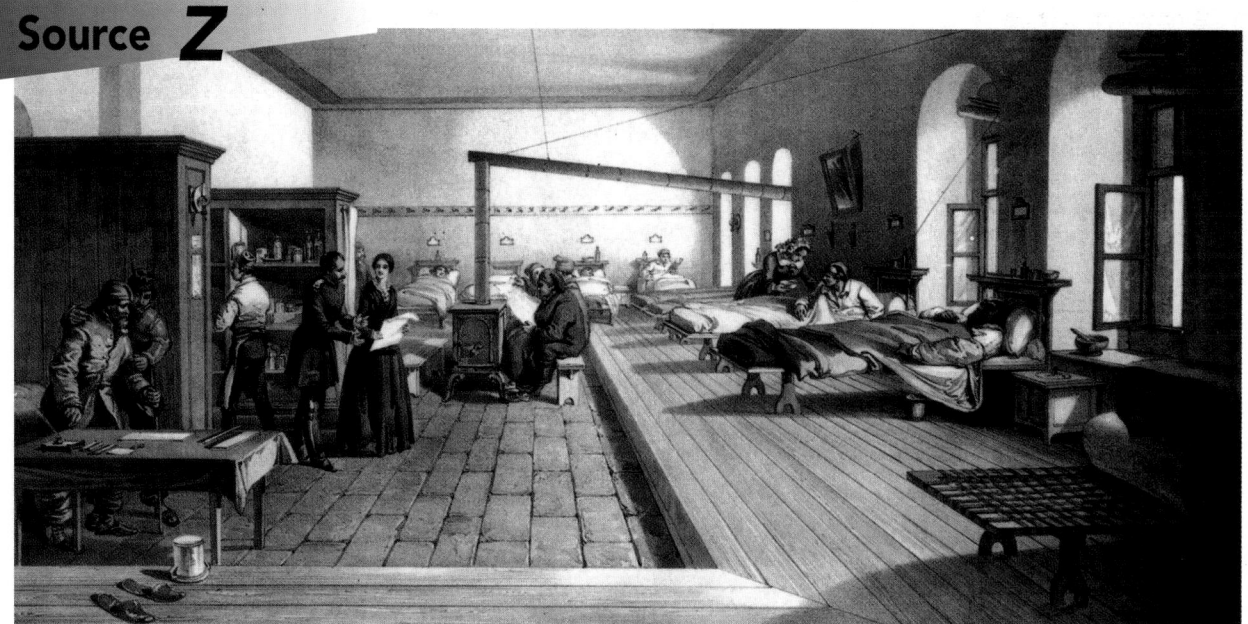

Nursing becomes a profession

Florence Nightingale returned to England and immediately won huge public acclaim. *The Times*, however, commented: 'While the benevolent deeds of Florence Nightingale are being handed down to posterity... are the human actions of Mrs Seacole to be entirely forgotten?' (24 November 1856). Nightingale had high hopes that her success in the Crimea would enable her to establish nursing as a respected profession. In 1859 she published a book called *Notes on Nursing* which described her methods. It stressed the importance of professionalism and ward hygiene and became the standard text for trainee nurses.

A public fund was opened to enable Nightingale to develop the training of nurses. It raised £44,000 and the money was used to start up the Nightingale School of Nursing at St Thomas's Hospital in London. It was here that the standards were laid down for the training of nurses. Trainees had to be disciplined and willing to work hard. They served a one-year probationary period and then trained for a further two years in order to qualify. Other training schools followed her example and, by 1900, there were 64,000 trained nurses in Britain.

▲ **A ward in the military hospital at Scutari, after it had been cleaned and reorganized by Nightingale nurses.**

In 1919 the Registration of Nurses Act was passed which laid down the qualifications needed to enter nursing. Today men also choose nursing as a career and it remains a highly respected profession.

QUESTIONS

1 What were the personal qualities of Florence Nightingale and Mary Seacole?

2 What contribution did each woman make to the nursing of troops during the Crimean War?

3 Was the presence of both women welcomed by the British army? Explain your answer.

4 Which woman is more important in the development of nursing as a profession? Give reasons for your answer.

5 Was a strong personality the only factor in Nightingale's success? Explain your answer.

ELIZABETH GARRETT ANDERSON
(1836–1917)

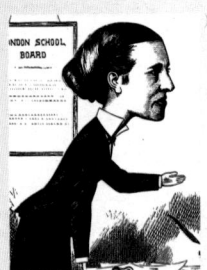

Having first worked as a nurse, Anderson tried to enter a medical school. From 1861–5 she applied to every college and hospital but was refused. Inspired by Elizabeth Blackwell she decided to fight the authorities and she succeeded in training privately. In 1865 she was accepted as a qualified doctor by the Society of Apothecaries and soon had a large practice in London.

SOPHIA JEX-BLAKE
(1840–1912)

Together with four other women, she gained entry to Edinburgh University in 1869 to study medicine. Their entry was deemed unlawful by the courts and they were dismissed from the course. She then founded the London School of Medicine for Women in 1874 and gained a medical degree from Bern University. She was the first female to set up a medical practice in Scotland.

In the mid-19th century women were not allowed to enter the universities. It was impossible, therefore, for them to obtain a degree in medicine and become practising doctors. In 1849 Elizabeth Blackwell, an American woman born in Britain, was awarded a medical degree by a New York college. In Britain most doctors fiercely opposed the entry of women into the medical profession, partly because they believed that women were 'too emotional' to do such important work.

In the 1860s there were signs of a change in society's attitude towards women. By this time, some men were also arguing that women should be emancipated (freed), allowed to vote, and have the same rights to education and a choice of work as men. Elizabeth Garrett Anderson and Sophia Jex-Blake (see boxes) were the first women to gain medical qualifications in Britain and, in doing so, pointed the way to future developments. Women made a vital contribution to the medical services in both the First and Second World Wars and by the mid-20th century, women had made significant progress in being accepted into the medical profession. In 1975 the passing of the Sex Discrimination Act meant that jobs were open to everyone, irrespective of whether they were male or female.

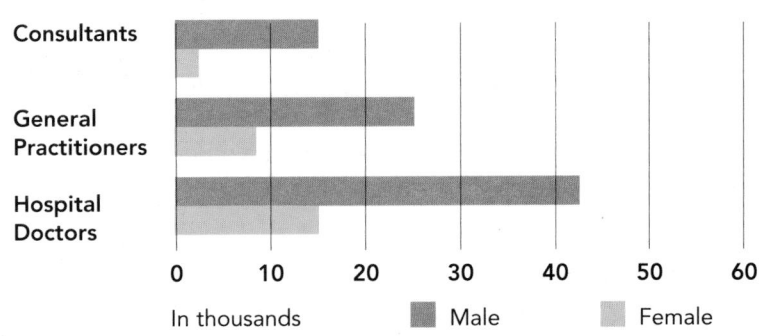

▲ Female doctors employed in the National Health Service in 1989. These statistics were published by the Department of Health.

QUESTIONS

1 What factors enabled women to progress in the medical profession?

2 What evidence is there here that there is still progress to be made?

12.6 Exercise

Source 1

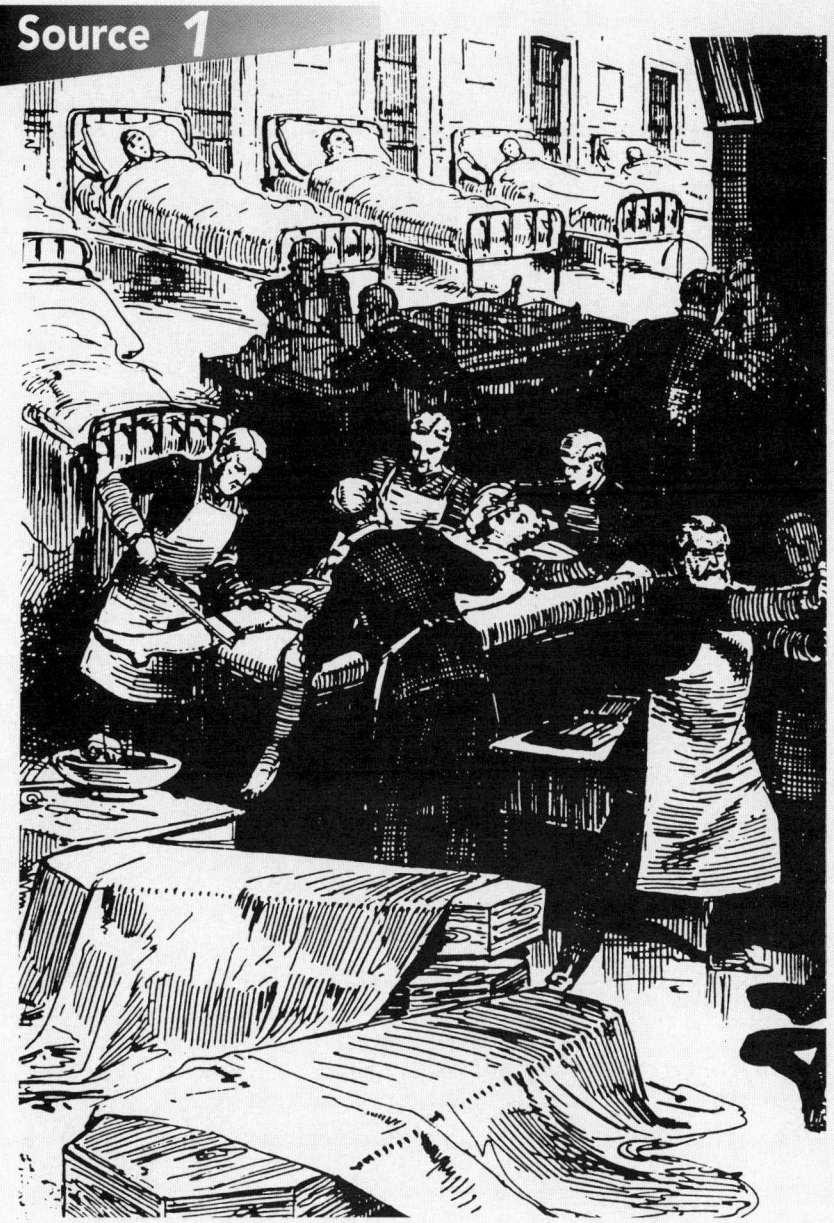

▲ 'Operation Madness', a cartoon from the 1870s. Anaesthetics came into general use at about this time.

Source 2

With the introduction of anaesthesia surgeons were free to try operations which before had been beyond them . . . There was some danger before the introduction of antiseptics that the risk of infection was increased.

▲ Richard Shryock, *The Development of Modern Medicine*, 1948.

Source 3

A system of washing is much better [than carbolic acid spray]. I fill the abdomen with warm water and wash all the organs. The water is plain unfiltered tap water and has not been boiled.

▲ Lawson Tait, a well known surgeon in 1882, describing how operations could be successfully carried out without using antiseptics.

(It may be helpful to look back through Chapters 11 and 12.)

1 Why did it take until the late 19th century for anaesthetics and antiseptics to be introduced widely into surgery?

2 'The introduction of anaesthetics and antiseptics was welcomed at the time'. Is this statement true?

3 Is Source 1 useful to historians studying operations in the 1870s?

4 Which do you think has contributed most to the development of surgery since 1850:
 • new machines
 • new scientific ideas
 • the growth of a nursing profession?
Give reasons for your answer.

CHAPTER 13

DEVELOPMENTS IN PUBLIC HEALTH

13.1 Public health up to 1850

Poor living conditions

The Industrial Revolution of the late 18th and early 19th century led to a rapid expansion of towns around the new factories in which the new machinery of the manufacturing industries were situated. Workers had to be near their place of work. An increasing number of people moved to towns. They had to accept living and working conditions which were very poor. Wages were low and people could not afford high rents. Some people lived in old buildings. Houses for the working class were built as cheaply as possible. There were no building or planning regulations. Little provision was made for the disposal of sewage or for getting fresh water, apart from communal wells. The government had a policy of *laissez-faire*. This means that they were not prepared to interfere into how people lived their lives, or into working and living conditions.

Town houses were often built on a back-to-back system. Sometimes they were built round a courtyard. These, like the roads, were unpaved and became muddy and contaminated with sewage. Houses were **verminous**, badly ventilated and overcrowded. Waste was piled in the courtyard or thrown into streams. Wells and watercourses quickly became polluted.

Industry made problems worse. Factory chimneys belched smoke and fumes into the air and their waste products polluted the rivers.

THE GROWTH OF TOWNS 1801–1901 (in thousands)			
City	1801	1851	1901
Birmingham	71	233	523
Bradford	13	104	280
Leeds	53	172	429
Liverpool	82	376	704
Manchester	70	303	645
Newcastle	33	88	247
Nottingham	29	57	240
Sheffield	46	135	407

Source A

Alfred and Beckwith Row consist of a number of buildings, each of which is divided into two houses, one back and the other front. These houses are surrounded by a broad open drain in a filthy condition. The houses have common, open privies [toilets] which are in the most offensive condition. In one house I found six persons occupying a very small room, two in bed, ill with fever. In the room above this were two more persons in one bed, ill with fever. In this same room a woman was carrying out the process of silk weaving.

▲ Living conditions in Bethnall Green, London, as described by Dr Thomas Southwood-Smith in 1838.

▼ A view of Manchester looking from the London and North-Western railway, about 1854.

Source B

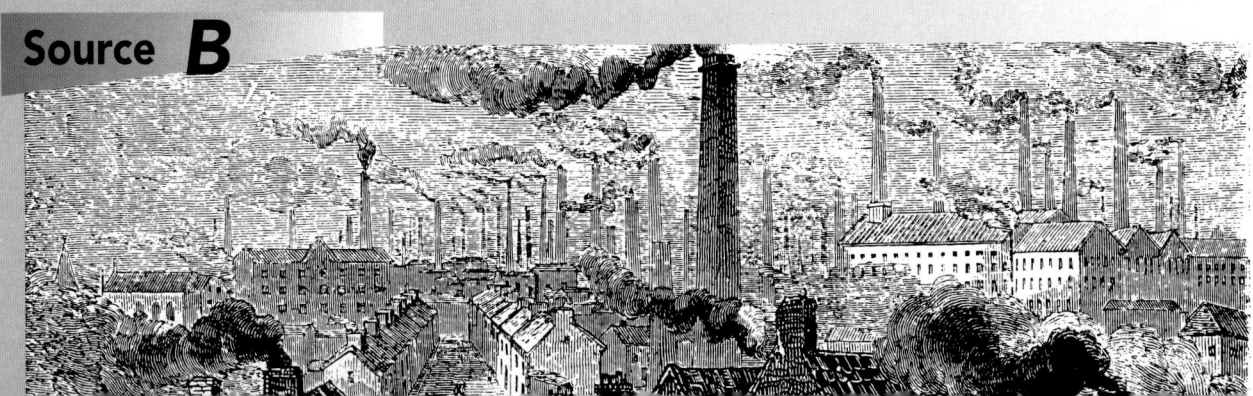

Disease

Bad living conditions meant that infectious diseases spread easily. The smallpox scourge of the 18th century was accompanied by tuberculosis, influenza and 'fever'. The fevers were typhoid, spread through dirty water, and typhus that was spread by the bites of body lice, which most people had because of poor personal hygiene.

These endemic diseases, which were always present in the population, were joined, in 1831–2, by a new epidemic, a disease which finally reached Britain and suddenly infected large numbers of people. This was cholera, which had been spreading across Europe from China and India since the beginning of the century.

Cholera is caused by a germ that attacks the intestines and leads to diarrhoea, vomiting, cramps, fever and death. The disease is spread through water that is infected by sewage from the victims. Cholera was first known to have entered Britain when William Sproat, a sailor, died in the port of Sunderland.

Doctors at the time had no idea what caused cholera or how to cure it. In some places barrels of tar were burnt in the streets to try to ward off 'poisonous miasmas', invisible gases that were thought to be the cause of disease. The disease spread rapidly and so many people died that the government was forced to act. Instructions were given about the immediate burial of the dead and the depth of burial.

By the end of 1832, most places in Britain had been affected by cholera and over 21,000 people had died. Then the disease seemed to die out and the boards of health that had been set up to combat it were abolished. Cholera was to return, however, in 1848, 1854 and 1866.

Source C

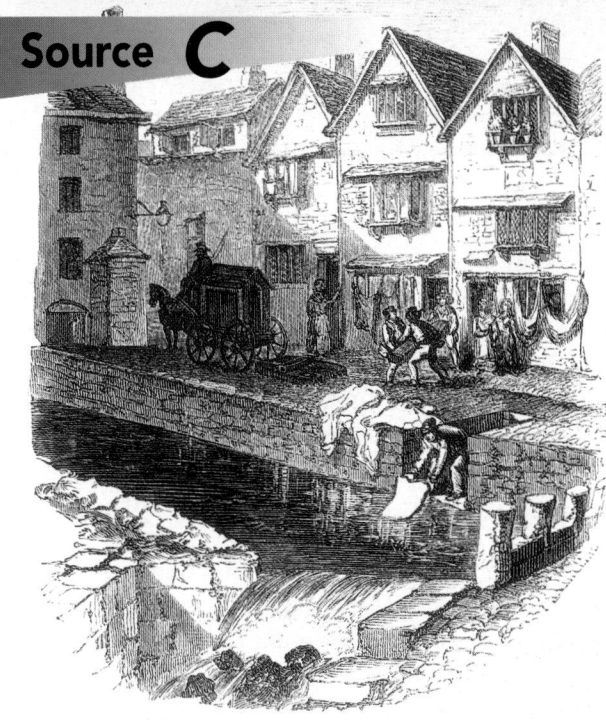

▲ Washing a cholera victim's bedclothes in the Mill Stream in Exeter, 1832. The stream being used was also the main source of drinking water for the city.

Source D

Dwellings are occupied by from five to fifteen families huddled together in dirty rooms. There are slaughter houses in Butcher Row with putrid heaps of offal. Pigs are kept in large numbers. Poultry are kept in cellars and outhouses. There are dung-heaps everywhere.

▲ From *The History of the Cholera in Exeter in 1832*, written by Dr Thomas Shapter, in 1841.

Source E

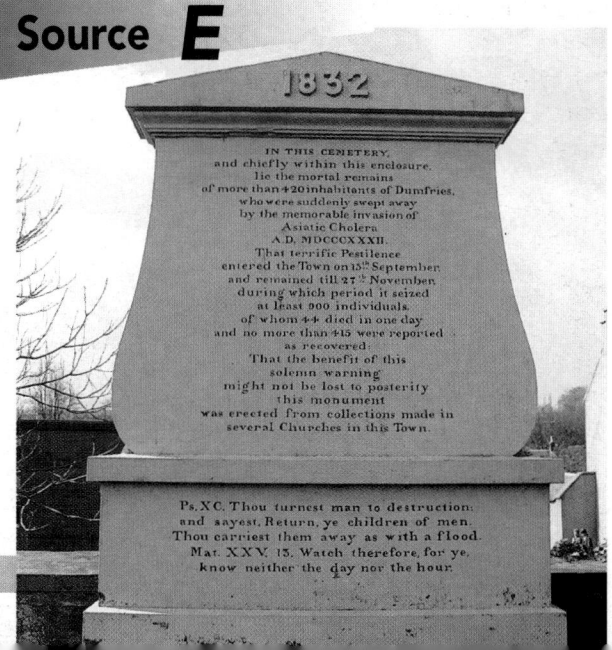

▶ A memorial to 420 cholera victims in Dumfries, Scotland, 1832.

Edwin Chadwick and public health

The crisis brought about by the cholera epidemic of 1832 prompted the government to act. Edwin Chadwick published the *Report on the Sanitary Condition of the Labouring Population of Great Britain* in 1842. It contained evidence from doctors involved in the workings of the **Poor Law** all over the country. The information it contained about the squalor in which many working people lived and worked shocked and horrified the wealthy classes. When taken together with statistics about birth and death compiled by William Farr, from 1839, a picture was built up that showed that something needed to be done about public health in Britain.

Chadwick was convinced that sickness was the cause of poverty. He was supported by the findings of Dr Southwood Smith who, in 1838, found 14,000 cases of fever among the poor of Whitechapel, London.

Source F

In one part of Market Street is a dunghill. Yet it is too large to be called a dunghill. I do not overestimate its size when I say that it contains 100 cubic yards [76 cubic metres] of impure filth which has been collected from all parts of the town. It is never removed. It is the main supply of a person who deals in dung. He sells it by the cart full. To please his customers he holds some back as the older the filth, the higher the price. The moisture oozes through the wall and over the pavement. This place is horrible, with swarms of flies which give a strong taste of the dunghill to any food left uncovered.

▲ A description of conditions in Greenock, Scotland, by Dr Laurie. It was included in Chadwick's 1842 Report to Parliament.

Source G

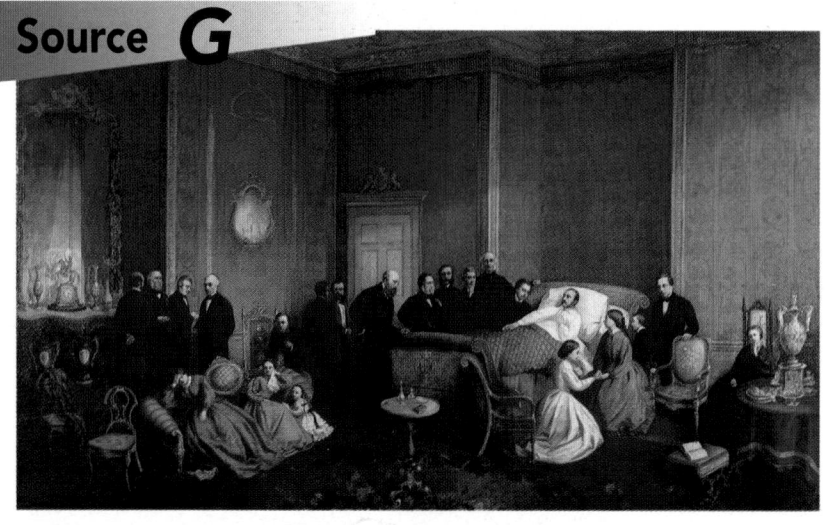

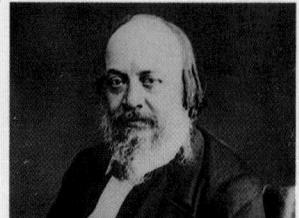

Chadwick believed that all laws should be useful and efficient. He first worked as a lawyer but, in 1832, he became a civil servant when he helped to investigate the Poor Laws. In 1838 he was given permission to inquire into the living conditions of the poor in the East End of London. In 1840 he began a national investigation of living conditions and, in 1842, published his *Report on the Sanitary Condition of the Labouring Population*. This revealed the terrible conditions in the towns and shocked the nation. Chadwick argued that if the towns were cleaner, there would be less disease and people would not need to take time off work. As a result, fewer people would need poor relief and this would save the ratepayers money. His work inspired the sanitary reform movement.

Chadwick said that Parliament should pass legislation to improve sewage disposal and water supplies. Although he was hard working and intelligent, Chadwick could often be argumentative and tactless. He was 'pensioned off' by the government in 1854.

◀ Not even the most privileged could escape disease. This painting, dating from about 1862, shows the last moments of Prince Albert, Queen Victoria's husband. He died of typhoid fever in 1861, caught from the drains of Windsor Castle.

The sanitary reform movement

Public health reform was slow to happen. Chadwick's 1842 report, however, did spark off a fierce debate about cleaning up the towns. Supporters of reform became known as the 'Clean Party'. In 1844 the Health of Towns Association was set up to campaign for healthier living conditions. Local branches of the Association were set up across the country. Each produced evidence of filthy streets, lack of sewage facilities and inadequate supplies of fresh water. The Association called for an Act of Parliament.

In 1847 a Public Health Bill was finally introduced into Parliament. It was strongly opposed by a group of MPs who were nicknamed the 'Dirty Party'. They believed in *laissez-faire* and argued that it was not the government's responsibility to clean up the towns. Furthermore, cleaning up the towns would cost too much money and make the government too powerful. The poor were often looked down on and it was thought they should try and help themselves. The poor did not have votes, so why should the wealthy try to help? Although Chadwick's report clearly showed that there was a connection between dirty living conditions and disease, no one knew exactly what caused these diseases.

Then, in 1848, cholera struck again and MPs voted in favour of the Bill which became the first Public Health Act.

Source H

Epidemic disease amongst the labouring classes is caused by atmospheric impurities produced by decomposing animal and vegetable substances, by damp and filth, and overcrowded dwellings. The annual loss of life is greater than the loss from death or wounds in any wars in modern times. The most important and practical measures are drainage, refuse removal and the improvement of water supplies. This expense would be a financial gain by lessening the cost of sickness and death. To prevent disease it would be efficient to appoint a district medical officer.

▲ Chadwick's main conclusions from the Report of 1842.

Source I

The chief theme of the speakers in opposition to the plan related to saving the pockets of the ratepayers. Their idea was calculated more to save an outlay of money than to ensure efficiency. The sewers were to discharge into the river nearby thus continuing the pollution.

▲ Opposition to a new sewerage scheme in Leeds described by James Smith in his *Report on the Condition of the Town of Leeds*, 1844.

The First Public Health Act 1848

Central Board of Health in London to sit for five years.

Local Boards of Health could be set up in towns if 10% of the rate payers agreed. These boards had the power to improve water supply and sewage disposals. They took over from private companies and individuals.

The Act was not compulsory. It was not fully applied across the whole country.

▲ The terms of the first Public Health Act, 1848.

QUESTIONS

1 What public health problems resulted from the Industrial Revolution?

2 What effects did the cholera epidemic of 1831–2 have?

3 What motives did Edwin Chadwick have for trying to improve public health?

4 Why was there opposition to reform during the 1840s?

5 Why was the first Public Health Act eventually passed in 1848?

The impact of the 1848 Public Health Act

The 1848 Act brought only limited improvements. Under the Act, local health boards, were set up in only 182 towns. As a result, sewage disposal and water supplies were improved in some of these places.

In 1854 those who were opposed to the Central Board of Health in London, were able to bring it to an end. Many water companies, landlords and builders had hated its very existence. Others still firmly believed that it was wrong for the government to interfere in people's private lives. *The Times* said, 'We prefer to take our chance of cholera and the rest than be bullied into health'. There was also bad feeling between Edwin Chadwick and the medical profession. Chadwick thought that preventing the environment from becoming filthy was the key to a healthy nation. Thus, he emphasized the need for clean water supplies and good sanitation. He did not appreciate that curative measures such as good doctors and hospitals also had a part to play. Meanwhile in September 1854, Dr John Snow had deduced that water was responsible for the spread of cholera when he plotted the victims of the disease in Broad Street, London, and found they used water from the same local pump. He removed the handle of the pump and the disease disappeared. In 1858 public health came under the control of the Privy Council and Sir John Simon, a surgeon, was made the Medical Officer of Health. He believed that public health involved both preventative and curative measures.

Further government measures

By the mid 1860s, the government realized that it would have to become more consistently involved in providing public health. A number of factors brought about this change of attitude (see diagram).

In 1869 Simon persuaded the government to set up the Royal Sanitary Commission. It found that the provision of clean water was still very patchy and recommended that laws should be made which were 'uniform, universal and imperative'. The government responded by forming the Local Government Board (1871) to oversee the administration of public health. The 1872 Public Health Act divided the country into 'sanitary areas' each with a medical officer of health. In 1875 Benjamin Disraeli's Conservative government passed a second Public Health Act and the Artisans' Dwellings Act – which together formed the most wide-reaching legislation to date.

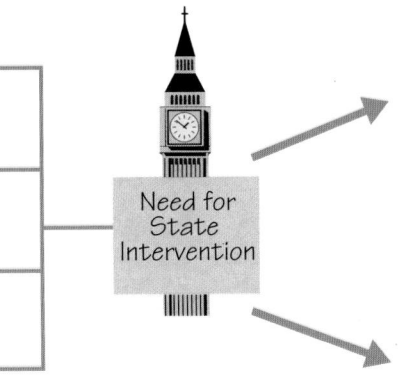

- Further cholera outbreaks in 1854 and 1866 frighten the authorities once more.
- In 1854 Dr John Snow showed that cholera was spread by contaminated water.
- In 1864 Louis Pasteur demonstrated the germ theory of disease. Need for cleanliness became clear.
- By the 1870s statistics showed that poor living conditions and disease were connected.

Need for State Intervention

1875 Second Public Health Act

- brought together all previous laws under one act.
- councils compelled to provide street lighting, clean water, drainage, and sewage disposal.
- councils had to employ medical inspectors.

1875 Artisans' Dwellings Act

- councils given power to buy up areas of slum housing, knock them down and build new houses.
- few councils took advantage.

▲ **Factors leading to state intervention into public health.**

The work of the Liberals 1906–14

In 1906 the Liberals won the general election with a massive majority. Many Liberal politicians, including David Lloyd George and Winston Churchill, stated that it was time for the government to tackle the social evils present in society. There were a number of reasons for this change in attitude.

Between 1886 and 1903 Charles Booth, a shipowner and social investigator, carried out a survey into living conditions in the East End of London. He published his findings in *Life and Labour of the People* in London. Booth concluded that about one-third of the people lived on incomes lower than 21s (£1.05) per week. In his opinion this was below the poverty line. They lived in sub-standard housing and had a poor diet. If they fell ill they could not afford to pay a doctor. In 1899 Seebohm Rowntree, a member of the chocolate manufacturing family, conducted his own inquiry in York. And his findings were very similar. Booth said that poverty was caused by sickness, old age, low wages and lack of employment – not laziness and drunkenness as many believed. There were no old age pensions. Old people who could not support themselves had only the workhouse to turn to. Many skilled workers could afford to pay into Friendly Societies and insure themselves against unemployment and illness. Unskilled workers, however, could not afford the subscriptions.

In 1902 the nation was shocked to find that 40 per cent of those that had volunteered to fight in the **Boer War** were suffering from malnutrition and diseases such as rickets, caused by poor diet. It was clear ill-health was linked to poverty and that government action was needed to raise living standards. Some Liberal MPs were concerned that people would vote for the newly formed Labour Party if they did not help the poor.

The Liberals went on to pass a wide range of reforms (see diagram). Churchill said, 'Our cause is the cause of the left out millions. We are all agreed that the state must concern itself with the care of the sick, the aged and, above all, children.'

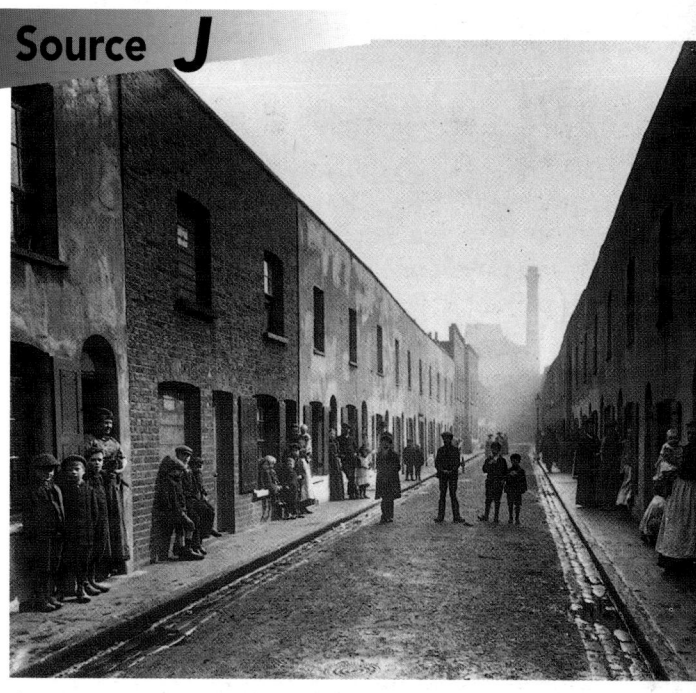

Source J

▲ Slum housing in the east end of London in 1912.

Date	Legislation
1906	**Provision of school meals** – local authorities given the power to provide free school meals.
1907	**School medical inspections.**
1909	**Old Age Pension Act** – people over 70 to receive 5s [25p] per week state pension as long as their income from other sources was not more than 12s [60p] per week.
1909	**Labour Exchanges** set up to help unemployed find work.
1911	**National Insurance Act** – two parts: Part I: Workers in manual trades earning less than £160 per year to pay 4d [2p] per week. The employer added 3d [1½p] and the government 2d [1p]. Workers entitled to 10s [50p] per week if they were off work sick, for up to 26 weeks. Free medical treatment available from a panel doctor. Part II: Workers, earning less than £160 per year in certain trades, together with the government and employers paid in 2½d [1p] per week. Workers could claim 7s [35p] unemployment pay for up to 15 weeks.

▲ Social reforms of the Liberal government 1906–14.

How did people react to the reforms?

For the first time the state had made a co-ordinated attack on poverty. Much of the legislation, however, was not very far-reaching and Lloyd George admitted that they had only just made a start. Nevertheless there was fierce resistance to some of the measures.

To pay for old age pensions, Lloyd George introduced the People's Budget, that aimed to tax the rich to provide for the poor. The House of Lords, largely made up of wealthy landowners, refused to pass the budget. This issue forced two general elections in 1910. The Liberals were narrowly returned. The budget was then allowed through but, in 1911, the power of the House of Lords to throw out finance bills was abolished by the Parliament Act. The Labour Party said that pensions should have been payable at 65, whereas many Conservatives were of the opinion that pensions 'would profoundly weaken the moral fibre of the nation, (report in *The Times*, 17 December 1909). People who qualified for a pension, however, were thankful to 'Lord' George.

The National Insurance Act was also widely condemned. Friendly societies and private insurance companies said that they would lose business. To overcome this, Lloyd George agreed to drop proposals for pensions to be paid to orphans and widows. He also allowed the Act to be administered by private insurance companies acting as 'approved societies' on behalf of the government. The Labour Party said that workers should not have to pay any money at all into the scheme, arguing that benefits should be paid entirely from taxes. Many doctors opposed the Act. They now had to register with a panel (a local list) and would receive 6 shillings (30p) for each patient under their care. Doctors argued that this meant a loss of independence and would cause medical standards to drop. In the face of such opposition, Lloyd George had to be strong and prepared to negotiate.

Government and social welfare 1919–39

After the First World War (1914–18) Lloyd George, by now the Prime Minister, promised to make Britain 'a country fit for heroes to live in'.

In 1919 the Ministry of Health was set up to administer all matters to do with health. This, in itself, was an important step forward as previously health came under the jurisdiction of seven different government departments. During the war, house building had been neglected so, in 1919, the new Minister for Health, Christopher Addison, passed the Housing and Town Planning Act. Under this Act the government gave local authorities a grant to help them build council houses. In 1920 the Unemployment Insurance Act extended insurance cover to all workers (except farm labourers and domestic servants) who earned less than £250 per year.

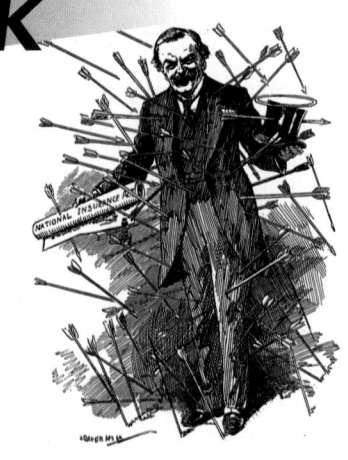

▲ Lloyd George had to overcome fierce opposition in steering the National Insurance Bill through Parliament. Do you think the cartoonist was a Lloyd George supporter?

QUESTIONS

1 Why was the Central Board of Health abolished in 1854?

2 Study the diagram on page 114. Which factor was the most important in bringing greater government involvement in public health?

3 Why did the Liberals pass a wide range of social reforms?

4 Summarize the main Acts passed by the Liberals under these headings:

 • Acts dealing with children
 • Acts dealing with the unemployed
 • Acts dealing with health and sickness
 • Acts dealing with the elderly.

5 The Liberal reforms helped many people. Why was there opposition to them at the time?

Rising unemployment

By 1922 the economy was in trouble. There was a slump in trade and rising unemployment. The government was forced to reduce its spending on housing, education and welfare provision. Other ways had to be found of funding reforms. Neville Chamberlain, Minister of Health from 1924–9, therefore encouraged the private sector to build more houses. The Pensions Act of 1925 was also Chamberlain's work. Pensions, funded by contributions from the state, employer and worker, were introduced at the age of 65. During the 1930s there was a world depression with mass unemployment. Dealing with the unemployed was more urgent than introducing welfare measures. The government was short of money and, therefore, reluctant to finance social reforms.

Despite this some progress in social provision was made between 1919 and 1939 (see Source M). The main problem was that the welfare services were an administrative muddle. Some services were provided by the government and some by private organizations. Health care, in particular, was a 'chaotic mixture' (see diagram). Opinion was growing that the health care system needed to be reformed. The Socialist Medical Association and the trade unions said that health services should be organized by the state. Others, however, still believed that voluntary organizations and self-help had a part to play. Many thought that social welfare should be provided only for the poor. It was argued that people who had the money should pay for their own medical treatment and schooling. The Second World War (1939–45) was to change many people's attitudes to welfare provision.

Source L

▲ This *Punch* cartoon from October 1937 portrays Neville Chamberlain as anxious to lead the way to health reforms. Chamberlain was Chancellor of the Exchequer from 1931–7. The reality was that the government was mainly concerned with the problem of unemployment caused by the depression.

An unco-ordinated system

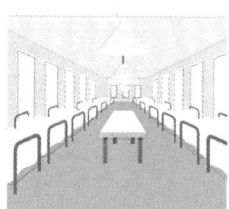

Hospitals
- About 3,000 in Britain, 1,000 were run by voluntary funds. Hospitals unevenly spread.
- Poor people were treated in workhouse infirmaries.

Doctors
- Wealthy received best treatment as they could afford the fees.
- Some workers, covered by National Insurance, had panel doctors. [dependants not covered]

Other services
Local authorities provided:
- school medical inspectors
- ante-natal clinics
- infant-welfare centres.

▲ Health care in 1939.

Source M

[In 1939] Britain was one of the most advanced of all countries in social provision. The majority of manual workers [but not their wives and children] were covered by social insurance schemes... The social services were complex and growing. State elementary schools and municipal hospitals were familiar landmarks. Ante-natal clinics and infant welfare centres were multiplying, and three million children received free milk in school.

▲ Paul Addison, *A New Jerusalem*, 1994.

The birth of the Welfare State 1945–51

In the early months of the war, children from the inner cities were evacuated to rural areas to escape the air raids. Many middle-class people were totally shocked at the filthy, deprived and badly clothed children who arrived in their towns and villages.

To cope with all the casualties caused by the air raids, the government set up the Emergency Medical Service. Hospitals were put under the Ministry of Health and free treatment was provided. This arrangement proved to be very successful.

In 1942 the Beveridge Report was published. It was the work of Sir William Beveridge, a leading civil servant. Beveridge recommended that the government should provide a welfare state by 'taking charge of social security from the cradle to the grave'. He argued that all citizens should have the right to be free from the five 'giants' of want, hunger, disease, ignorance, squalor and idleness. The Beveridge Report became a best seller and pointed the way to a better society after the war was over. People came to believe that the state had a responsibility to everyone, not just the poor. Members of all the political parties welcomed the Report but Winston Churchill spoke for many Conservatives when he argued that Beveridge's plan would be far too costly to implement.

The National Health Service

In July 1945 the Labour Party came to power, and it fell to them to introduce a Beveridge-style welfare state. **Family Allowances** and compulsory **National Insurance** for everyone was introduced in 1948. The central hub of Labour's reform programme was the National Health Service, masterminded by the Minister of Health, Aneurin Bevan. The NHS was to provide free medical treatment for everyone. It came into operation on 5 July 1948. Hospitals came under the control of the state and local authorities were to provide free services including ambulances, vaccination programmes, environmental health, maternity clinics and health visitors. Doctors, opticians and dentists provided a free service. The NHS was not welcomed by everyone. The BMA, which spoke for the doctors, was at first violently opposed to it. Doctors feared that the NHS would dictate to them where they had to practise and they would be given a fixed salary. There were many angry discussions between Charles Hill, the secretary of the BMA, and Aneurin Bevan. In the end Bevan won the doctors over by stating that they would be paid a fee for each patient they had registered and agreeing that they would be allowed to treat private fee-paying patients if they wished. By June 1948, 92 per cent of doctors and the vast majority of hospitals had agreed to work under the NHS.

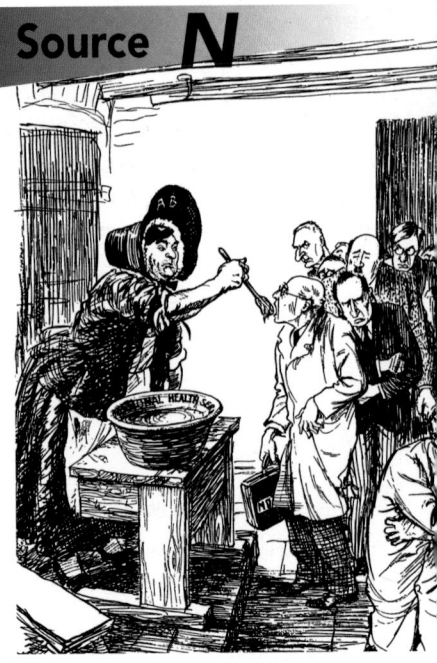

▲ Bevan dishes out NHS 'medicine' to the doctors. Many doctors were opposed to the NHS at first.

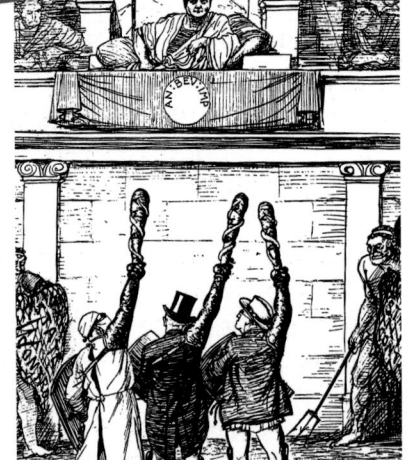

MORITURI TE SALUTANT

▲ A *Punch* cartoon from 1948. The Latin words mean: 'We who are about to die, salute you.' This was often said to the Emperor by gladiators in Roman times.

Reactions to the NHS

The NHS was received with enthusiasm by most people. Immediately, people took advantage of the free medical services. By 1950 the NHS was costing the government £350m per year, over twice the figure predicted. In 1950 the government was faced with financing the armed forces in the Korean War. Prescription charges were introduced, along with other tax increases, and this prompted the resignation of Aneurin Bevan.

The Introduction of Free Vaccinations in Britain	
1840	Smallpox
1948	Tuberculosis
1954	Diphtheria, whooping cough and tetanus ('triple vaccine')
1955	Polio
1964	Measles
1969	Rubella (German measles)

Vaccination programmes

After 1948 the drive to improve the population's personal health was stepped up. Vaccination programmes, funded by the state, were put in place for all children (see box). In 1954 Jonas Salk produced an effective vaccine against polio, a terrifying disease which, at its worst, could cause paralysis; it struck particularly at young people. In 1960 Albert Sabin produced an improved vaccine which could be taken orally on a sugar lump.

In 1948 the World Health Organization (WHO), an agency of the United Nations, was set up. One of its aims is to encourage vaccination programmes on a world-wide basis. Advances have been made and today eight out of every ten children have been vaccinated against the major killer diseases. It is hoped that by the year 2000, 90% of the world's children will have been immunized.

Alternative medicine

There has been a re-emergence of alternative treatments for illness. Some people do not like modern drugs; they fear that they may have side-effects. A recent survey revealed that patients suffering from illnesses like stress, depression, chronic back pain, arthritis and eczema had benefited greatly from sessions with faith healers. Other natural treatments such as homeopathy and acupuncture may become available on the NHS.

Source P

She went and got tested for new glasses, then she went to the chiropodist, she had her feet done. Then she went back to the doctor's because she'd be having trouble with her ears and the doctor said he would fix her up with a hearing aid.

▲ How one old lady reacted to the NHS, quoted in Paul Addison, *Now the War is Over*, 1985.

Source Q

The Times warned its readers that there was a danger of Britain becoming a 'Santa Claus State'. Citizens might also get so used to having things served up on a plate that they would no longer try to help themselves.

▲ R. J. Cootes, *The Welfare State*, 1970.

Source R

When the NHS started, oh it was fantastic. My mother and dad had been having problems with their teeth for ages, and I think they were first at the dentist, as soon as he opened. And instead of having just a few teeth out they had the complete set out. And free dentures. Thought it was wonderful.

▲ A woman describing her reaction to the NHS.

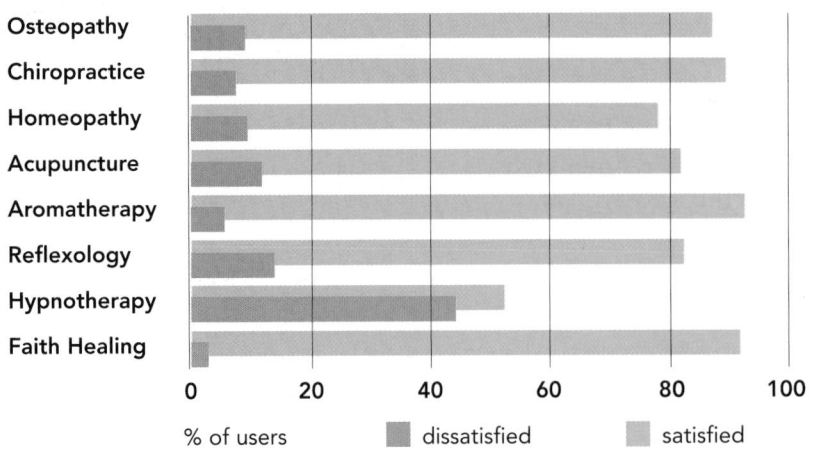

Osteopathy
Chiropractice
Homeopathy
Acupuncture
Aromatherapy
Reflexology
Hypnotherapy
Faith Healing

% of users   ■ dissatisfied   ■ satisfied

▲ **The results of a recent survey by the consumer magazine, *Which*. It shows that people who had tried alternative treatments mainly regarded them as successful.**

The NHS and change

Financing the NHS has proved to be a headache for successive governments. The cost is increased by the fact that the death rate has declined and people are living longer. Fierce political debates have taken place over the last twenty years about how to finance the NHS. Margaret Thatcher, the Conservative Prime Minister from 1979–90, encouraged the growth of private health insurance as a means of taking some of the pressure off the NHS. Critics of this policy, however, said it was creating a two tier system, with NHS patients receiving inferior treatment. Recently hospitals have been given control of their own budgets in an attempt to make the NHS cost effective. However, this has sometimes led to treatment being refused either because of lack of money or the fact that the illness was 'self-inflicted' (for example, illnesses related to smoking). This has caused outrage in some quarters. The NHS, however, has been a success and is held in high regard by many people.

QUESTIONS

1 Some historians have argued that the momentum for social reform started by the Liberal Government was lost between 1919 and 1939. Do you agree with this view?

2 What part did the following factors play in the introduction of a welfare state after 1945:
 • the work of the Liberal Government, 1906–14
 • changing social attitudes
 • the 1942 Beveridge Report
 • Labour's election victory in 1945?

3 Explain the reactions of ordinary people to the setting up of the NHS.

4 What changes have taken place in the NHS since 1950?

5 Is the increase in use of alternative medicine an example of change or continuity in the history of medicine? Explain your answer.

SUMMARY

▶ In the late 19th century the idea of *laissez-faire* was gradually abandoned. The government started to take more responsibility for public health.

▶ The Liberals passed a range of social reforms between 1906 and 1914, including the Old Age Pensions Act (1908) and the National Insurance Act (1911).

▶ Some welfare measures were passed between 1919 and 1939 but the government was preoccupied with the problem of mass unemployment.

▶ The Second World War (1939–45) helped to change attitudes towards social welfare. In 1942 the Beveridge Report recommended the formation of a welfare state.

▶ The National Health Service and compulsory National Insurance were introduced by the Labour Government of 1945–51.

▶ Changing social conditions in the late 20th century have resulted in a reappraisal of the way the NHS is organized.

Source 1

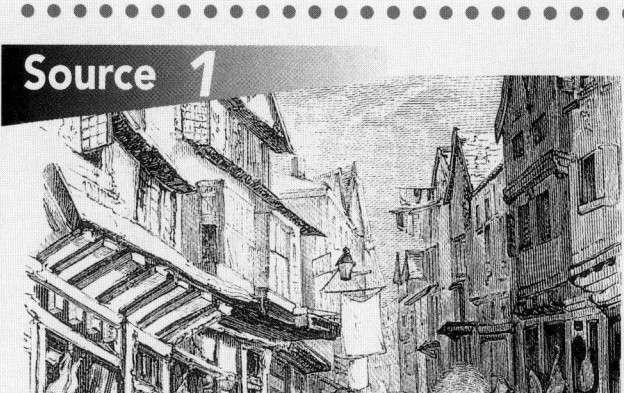

▲ Barrels of tar being burned in the streets of Exeter as a remedy for cholera, during the epidemic of 1831–2.

1 Burning barrels of tar will not stop diseases like cholera from spreading. Why, then, did many town councils order this to be done during the cholera epidemic of 1831–2?

2 Why were there four outbreaks of cholera between 1831 and 1866?

3 The first Act of Parliament to tackle the problems of public health effectively was the Public Health Act of 1875 (Source 3). Why was this Act so long delayed?

4 Which of the events shown in Source 3 did the most to bring about a Welfare State in Britain? Explain your answer

Source 2

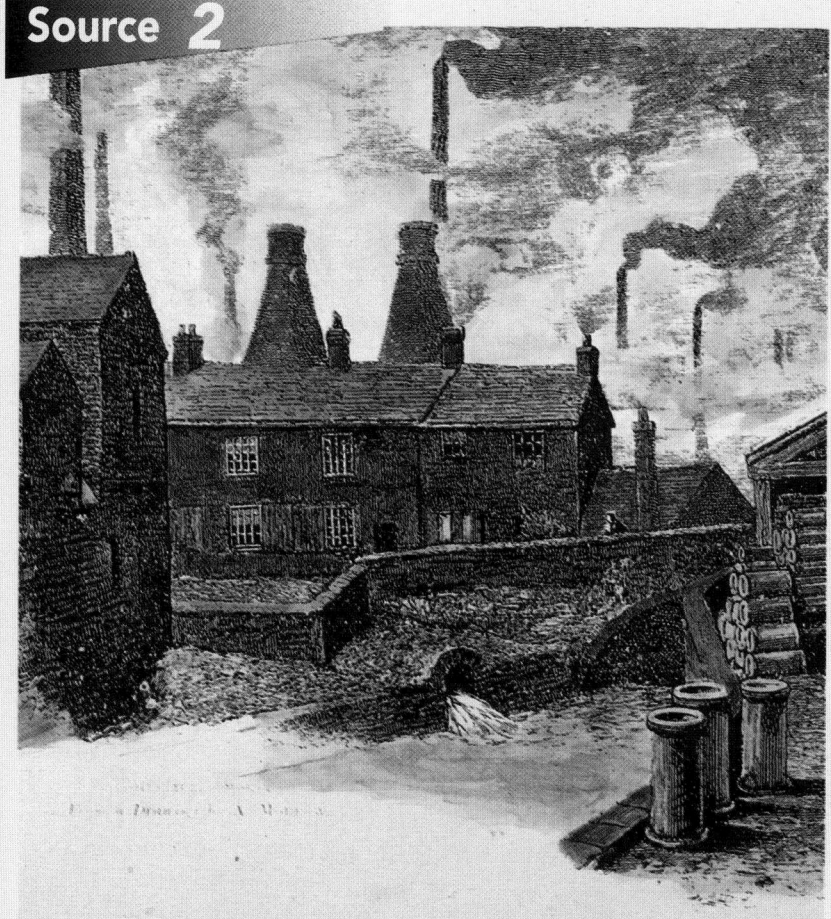

▲ A view of industrial Sheffield in the mid-19th century.

Source 3

Some events which improved health and welfare in Britain

1875 Second Public Health Act passed. Local councils were made to provide fresh water and sanitation.

1909 The first old age pensions were paid.

1942 The Beveridge Report said that the government should look after its citizens from 'the cradle to the grave'.

1948 The National Health Service came into being – free medical care for everyone.

▲ From a modern history book.

CHAPTER 14

Conclusion

14.1 Change

As we have now seen, the history of medicine is not one of steady progress. It is a story where the rate of change varies. At some times change was very rapid, at others very slow. Sometimes things changed for the better, at other times they got worse. It is not very useful to talk about medicine as a whole most of the time, either. We have looked at different aspects of medicine through time:

- *Understanding about the cause and cure of disease*
- *Anatomy*
- *Surgery*
- *Public health and prevention of disease*
- *Surgeons, doctors and nurses – the development of a medical profession.*

These different aspects of medicine have developed at different rates. For example, the standards of public health provision in British towns at the height of the Roman Empire was probably better than it was from the fall of the Empire until 1850, yet Graph A opposite (which looks at understanding of the cause and cure of disease) shows that in this aspect standards were higher from the middle of the 16th century onwards than in Roman times.

Understanding of the cause and cure of disease

Graph A tries to show how understanding of the cause and cure of disease rose and fell during the period we are studying. It is an interpretation, not a fact. Each 50 years has been given a mark out of 10 to represent 'standards'. There are many assumptions built into it, the most important is that we are comparing the best practice being used at each date.

The assumptions about the history of medicine made while preparing the graph are:

1 There was notable progress in Greece around the time of Hippocrates.
2 There was then very gradual improvement through to the late Roman Empire.
3 There was a sharp fall in standards during the Dark Ages.
4 This was followed by a slow rise in standards, which got faster following the establishment of medical schools in the Middle Ages.
5 There was another fast improvement during the Renaissance.
6 This was followed by a further period of gradual improvement until the discovery of the germ theory.
7 Since the acceptance of the germ theory our knowledge has increased rapidly with the identification of disease-causing microbes, and the development of vaccines and drugs.

The graph shows the rate of change – the faster the rate of change the steeper the gradient of line. It also suggests places where turning points occurred. The turning points are those places where there is a sharp change in angle.

Graph B, which shows standards in surgery, shows a pattern which is broadly similar, but different in some points of detail.

First of all the time period over which the graph has been plotted is slightly different. This is because we know something about prehistoric surgery. We do not know why trephining operations were performed, but we do know that they were and that many people survived.

Whereas the cause and cure graph starts with the standard achieved in Egypt immediately before the rise of the Greek civilization the surgery graph shows the improvements made by the Egyptians. It also shows a smaller improvement through Greek and Roman civilization relative to the standards achieved by the Egyptians than the cause and cure graph.

The two graphs follow a similar pattern until the Early Modern period when the cause and cure one shows a faster improvement than surgery. This pattern is reversed in the 19th century when the surgery graph shows faster progress before the cause and cure graph, reflecting the development of anaesthetics before the development of germ theory.

Try plotting your own graphs for
● public health
● anatomy
● the training of nurses and doctors.

Would you expect your new graphs to show a similar pattern to either of these?

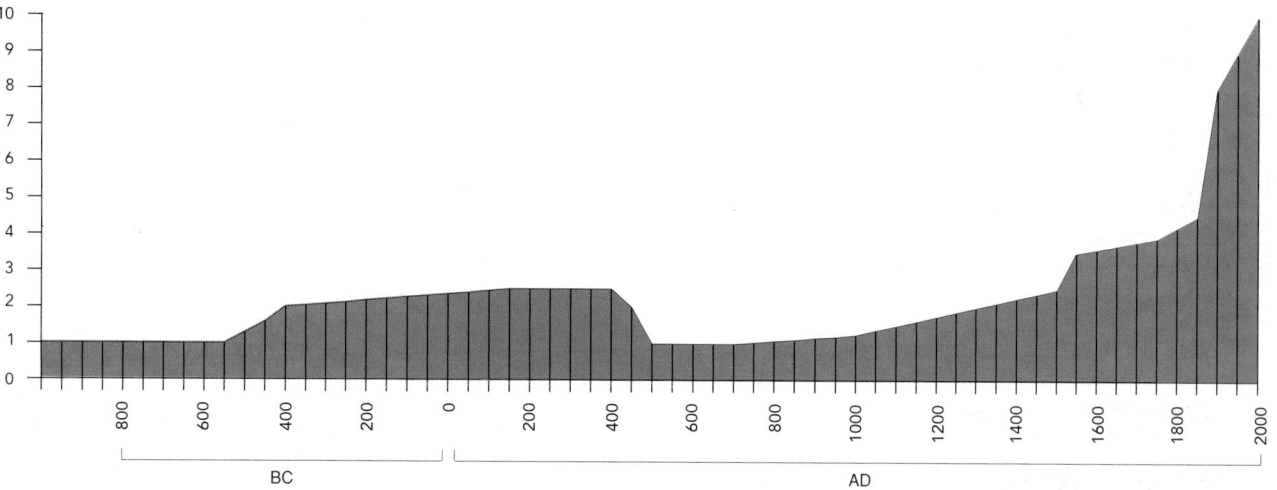

▲ Graph A: Standards in understanding of the cause and cure of disease.

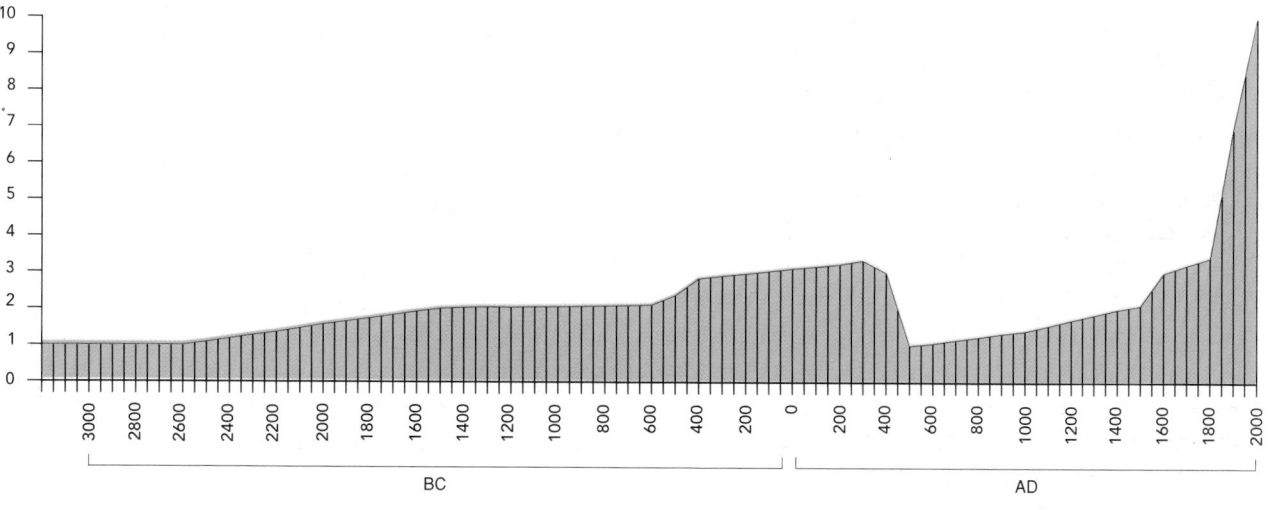

▲ Graph B: Standards in surgery.

Throughout your study of the history of medicine you have been using factors and concepts to help you understand what happened and why. The history of medicine presents you with an enormous amount of information. Factors and concepts give you the tools to shape this information into patterns.

In the exam you will often be set questions which concentrate on factors or concepts, not on particular people or events. The secret of success is to be able to show that you understand the factors and concepts, and that you can support your answers with examples taken from the history of medicine. Galen insisted the study of anatomy had to start with bones – he said they were like poles in tents. In a good exam answer the factors and the concepts are the bones, they give it shape, but the facts you use to support them are the organs and muscles, without which you have nothing but a skeleton of an answer.

Concepts

The table on this page deals with the most important concepts:

Development and change: where the distinction is between a new idea that builds on work that has gone before, or one which strikes off in different directions.

Progress and regress: where things can either get better or worse.

The rate of change: which is variable – sometimes things change very quickly, and other times very slowly or not at all.

Trends and turning points: trends take place over a long time and are made up of a number of related developments. Turning points are sudden changes which produce a change in direction.

Copy and complete the table below.
The table divides medicine into three time periods. **Ancient** (up to the end of the Roman Empire) **500–1800**, and **Modern** (from 1800 onwards). You need to find examples of each of the concepts in the left-hand column to fill in the gaps. The same example could be used to illustrate more than one point – germ theory is both progress and a turning point – but try to find as many different examples as you can.

	Ancient	500–1800	Modern
Progress			Discovery of blood groups leading to blood transfusion.
Regress			
Development			
Rate of change	Slow: the prehistoric period		
Trend		Belief that the planets and the zodiac affected a patient's health.	
Turning Point			

Factors

Factors and concepts do not work in isolation from each other. You can find a whole range of factors working with each concept. For example:

Chance: this can be seen to have been a key factor in bringing about both progress and regress. Chance caused regress when the Minoan civilization of Crete was destroyed and the advances the Minoans had made in sanitation and drainage were lost to the Mediterranean world. Chance was an equally important factor in progress when Paré ran out of boiling oil to use on gunshot wounds after a battle in 1537. He was forced to try a new treatment, which he would not otherwise have tried, and found it worked much better than the treatment with boiling oil. Both these cases illustrate chance – nobody planned that these events should happen, or decided they would be a good thing.

War: this can be shown to have speeded up the rate of change. The money put into medical development during the Second World War, and the new treatments developed under the pressure of the large numbers of casualties, resulted in changes from the mass-production of penicillin to the development of plastic surgery by Archibald McIndoe. Six years of war saw astonishing progress. War also had a negative effect on medicine. The collapse of the Roman Empire followed military defeat. This led to regress, most obviously in public health in most of Europe.

Religion: has also been a factor in both progress and regress. In the Middle Ages, from 1300 onwards, the Church had forbidden the boiling of bodies to produce skeletons for study by doctors and anatomists. The lack of knowledge about the skeleton this caused kept medieval anatomy below the standards that had been achieved by Galen and his contemporaries in the Roman Empire. Earlier, religion had helped medicine progress through the practice of mummification in Egypt which ensured doctors had some knowledge of human anatomy.

Copy and complete the chart below.

You may not be able to find an example for each slot in the table, but you should find you have a choice of many examples for some slots. Remember the best example is both a clear example of the influence of the factor, and has detailed factual support. In the exam you will get much more credit if your factual support is as detailed as possible.

	Progress	Regress	Development	Rate of Change	Trend	Turning Point
Chance	Paré developed treatment of wounds because he ran out of oil.	Destruction of Minoans meant knowledge of drainage etc lost				
War		Collapse of Roman public health system after military defeat.		Speeded up – McIndoe and mass-production of Penicillin, WW2.		
Religion	Mummification in Egypt increased knowledge of anatomy.	Church stopped study of skeletons in 1300, held back anatomy.				
Science & technology						
Communications						
Individuals						
Teamwork						

GLOSSARY

agar a jelly prepared from seaweed for bacteria to grow on for use in experiments.

AIDS Acquired Immune Deficiency Syndrome – a virus which attacks the immune system leaving the sufferer very open to infection.

antibody a defensive substance produced in the body to neutralize a foreign micro-organism or poison.

antibiotic drug derived from living organism, such as fungi, which would kill bacteria, or prevent it from growing.

antisepsis the use of antiseptics (first carbolic acid) to kill germs.

arsenic a chemical element which, though poisonous, is sometimes used in minute quantities in medicines.

ascendant the star or planet rising at the time of a person's birth.

asepsis sterilising the air, the clothing and tools of doctors in the operating room to remove the risk of germs.

astrology the study of the influence of the stars and planets on human events.

astronomy the study of stars, planets and other objects in space.

attenuation thinning something out or weakening it. Used in medicine to mean the idea of weakening a germ, so it loses its effectiveness.

bacillus any bacterium (microscopic plant) which causes disease.

barber-surgeons barbers who also performed minor surgery and dentistry. They were mainly used by the poor.

bezoar stone stony mass found in stomach of goats, antelopes, llama, etc., formally thought to be an antidote to all poisons.

Boer War a war fought in 1899–1902 between the small Dutch republics in South Africa and the British who saw all of South Africa as part of the British Empire.

caesarean section delivery of a child by cutting open the mother's abdomen.

caliph a Muslim leader during the time of the Islamic Empire.

cautery a method of treating amputated limbs or wounds by burning them with hot iron or oil to prevent infection and seal the wound.

Christendom all Christians.

circulating going round; Harvey's understanding of blood circulation was of enormous importance to medical development.

colycynth a kind of cucumber.

Crusades military expeditions in the name of Christianity to recover the Holy Land from Muslims.

distillation converting liquid into vapour by heating it and then condensing it again into droplets. This was done either to extract a component of the liquid or to purify it.

empirical relying on experience or observation.

Family Allowance an amount of money given weekly by the state for the support of children.

fibre optics extremely thin glass fibres which are used in optical instruments; their flexibility and use of maximum light make then ideally suited for use in very inaccessible places.

Islam the Muslim world.

immune resistant to disease.

National Insurance a system of compulsory insurance, paid for by weekly contributions by employers and employees, to pay for benefits to the sick, retired and unemployed.

Nationalism the belief in striving after the unity, independence, interests or domination of a nation.

natural something which is physical, observable and of this world.

opium a drug derived from the white poppy producing sleepiness, numbness, euphoria or loss of memory.

organic derived from a plant or animal organism.

pilgrimage a journey to a shrine or holy place.

plague there are two main forms of plague: bubonic (characterised by buboes or lumps), spread by flea bites; and pneumonic (respiratory), spread by coughing or sneezing.

Poor Law laws relating to the support of the poor.

progress moving forward, often implying improvement.

rational ruled by reason.

regress going backwards, often implying getting worse.

Renaissance rebirth; marked the transition from medieval to modern history beginning in the 14th century; a period when the arts and science flourished.

scarlet fever a contagious disease where the patient becomes feverish and their skin and the inside of the mouth and throat go bright red

solid cultures experimentally grown bacteria in nutritive solid substances.

sublimation purifying a substance by changing it from solid to vapour without passing through the liquid state (and usually back to solid) .

supernatural outside the world as we know it, sometimes involving gods, spirits and unknown forces.

suture a surgeon's stitch.

thalidomide a drug, withdrawn in 1961 because it was found to cause malformation in the foetus if taken during pregnancy.

tracheotomy an operation which involves cutting into the trachea or windpipe.

verminous to be infested with obnoxious insects such as, fleas and lice, and troublesome animals such as mice or rats.

INDEX